Praise for
The Mother-Daughter Puzzle

"If you've ever wanted to understand yourself better and enhance all of your important relationships then look no further than *The Mother-Daughter Puzzle*. Rosjke illustrates beautifully the significance of how relationships between mothers and daughters impact how we live, how we feel, how we love, and the world we live in... Stunning."

SERENA SIMMONS
Chartered Psychologist, Senior Lecturer
in Psychology, Nottingham Trent University,
Founder of Ape-Model Psychology

"Rosjke Hasseldine has unique insights into the complex, hidden, and deep-rooted dynamics of mothers and daughters. This book enables readers to understand many of the generational issues, values, traditions, and personality variables that impact the mother-daughter relationship. The *Mother-Daughter History Mapping* tool helps women to sensitively examine their inherited emotional patterns and behaviors. *The Mother-Daughter Puzzle* is an important resource that energizes women to create greater joy, respect, and love."

LOIS A. HERMAN
Coordinator, Women's UN Report Network

With love
Rosjke

"Bravo, Rosjke, for bringing our attention to this highly neglected area. This book is a must-read for all counselors and psychotherapists."

LORNA MARCHANT
Honorary Fellow, British Association for
Counselling and Psychotherapy

"*The Mother-Daughter Puzzle* provides a beautiful roadmap to healing and forgiveness between mothers and daughters."

GAYLE KIRSCHENBAUM
Emmy Award-winning filmmaker of
Look At Us Now, Mother!

"This highly anticipated book is essential reading for professional women who will benefit from learning how explicit and implicit messages from our earliest role models affect the choices we make as we take on (or don't) the leadership roles that greatly need our talents. As the foremost expert in this area, Rosjke provides valuable ideas about how to sort out lessons from our past and apply those that support our own unique aspirations."

VANESSA DRUSKAT, PHD
Associate Professor of Organizational Behavior,
Peter T. Paul College of Business & Economics,
University of New Hampshire

"This is a groundbreaking book with huge potential for further research. It fills a gap in academic research on women's empowerment by exploring the 'from-within' perspective. The author does not only unpack the poorly understood mother-daughter relationship, but also provides much-needed solutions."

FATIMA SADIQI, PHD
Woodrow Wilson Global Fellow, Professor of Linguistics and Gender Studies, Sidi Mohamed Ben Abdellah University, Author of *Moroccan Feminist Discourses*

"This engrossing book takes us beyond the surface level with stirring stories and insightful connections between mother-daughter relationship conflict and how women are treated in society."

SUSAN NEWMAN MANFULL, PHD
Social Psychologist, Creator of Provence WineZine & The Modern Trobadors

"Thank you, Rosjke, for the work you do and for a potent and humane response to the mother question. *The Mother-Daughter Puzzle* is a much-needed voice for women's rights and mothers' rights."

VANESSA OLORENSHAW
Author of *Liberating Motherhood*

"In *The Mother-Daughter Puzzle,* Rosjke Hasseldine provides a desperately needed revolution in our approach to dealing with generational conflict and the habitual patterns of self-sacrifice in women. Through deconstructing the causes of 'mother-blaming,' she shows us how inherited sexism is at the root of mother-daughter conflicts. In doing so, she provides a path forward for profound healing, not only of the mother-daughter relationship, but also for how we relate to the world as women."

AMY SEDGWICK
Cofounder, Red Tent Sisters

"I often wondered why I struggle with confidence at different phases of my career. Rosjke's *Mother-Daughter History Mapping* exercise helped me to recognize that this is directly linked to my choice of a path untraditional to all female generations in my family. My work with Rosjke has helped me to see myself and my mother in a completely new, more tender light."

TERI HULL
Chef and Health Coach

"*The Mother-Daughter Puzzle* skillfully unravels the complicated dynamics of the mother-daughter relationship schism. It explains how generational, cultural, and social ideologies have been imprinted on this highly important relationship and it provides a pathway to repair the mother-daughter bond."

JENNIFER PRICE
Founder, A Natural State of Being

"I cried when I read these stories, because they are mine, too. I personally know the power of solving *The Mother-Daughter Puzzle*, and am so heartened that all women now have access to this powerful, healing work from a woman I know as my personal therapist and inspiration."

STEPHANIE CLARK CIRIHAL
Evolutionary Love Coach

"A deeply empowering tool, this book helps us to recognize and break through inherited patterns of mother-daughter relationships—and what results is the freedom to change the paradigm in which we thought we had to live. Rosjke is inspiring change in womankind, one mother-daughter relationship at a time!"

ANTJE BOURDAGES
Spiritual Adviser, Founder, What's Behind Your Door

"*The Mother-Daughter Puzzle* brings stunning clarity to the role intergenerational dynamics play in what *isn't* working for women. An illuminating, lucid book that will change how you see yourself and your mom."

JENNIFER MAHER
Businesswoman

Books by Rosjke Hasseldine

The Silent Female Scream

The MOTHER-DAUGHTER *Puzzle*

A NEW GENERATIONAL UNDERSTANDING OF THE MOTHER-DAUGHTER RELATIONSHIP

ROSJKE HASSELDINE

Published by Women's Bookshelf Publishing

First published in Great Britain and the United States in 2017 by Women's Bookshelf Publishing
9 Surrey Lane, Durham, NH 03824, USA.

Library of Congress Cataloguing-in-Publication Data

Hasseldine, Rosjke
The mother-daughter puzzle: a new generational understanding of the mother-daughter relationship / Rosjke Hasseldine
p. cm.
ISBN 978-0-9557104-1-4 (Paperback)
ISBN 978-0-9557104-2-1 (Kindle)
1. Mothers and daughters. 2. Family relationships. 3. Women–Psychology. 4. Feminism. 5. Intergenerational relations. I. Hasseldine, Rosjke. II. Title.
HQ755.85.H37 2017
306.874'3—dc20

2017933339

The client stories in this book are fictional. They do not resemble actual people, living or dead. If you think you recognize yourself in these pages, this is entirely coincidental. The client stories reflect themes and issues with which many women struggle. The author's own stories represent her experiences and memories exclusively.

Please note that the author of this book does not dispense medical advice or prescribe the use of any technique as a form of treatment for physical, emotional, or medical problems without the advice of a physician, either directly or indirectly. The intent of the author is only to offer information of a general nature to help readers in their quests for emotional and spiritual wellbeing. In the event you use any of the information in this book for yourself, which is your constitutional right, the author and the publisher assume no responsibility for your actions or the outcome.

Author photo – Deborah Chaze
Cover artist – Tim O'Brien @ www.timobrienart.co.uk
Book Designer – Ingrid Paulson @ www.ingridpaulson.com

Printed, bound, and distributed by Lightning Source US

This book is dedicated to my daughter Olivia, my mother Tien, and my clients, in gratitude for all they have taught me about mothers and daughters.

CONTENTS

INTRODUCTION

When women are heard, mothers and daughters are able to listen to each other.

THE STORY OF how I came to write this book started a long time ago on an ordinary sunny day in Christchurch, New Zealand when I was sixteen. I had just returned to school after having been home for lunch and as I locked my bike to the bike stands, I heard a voice warn me I should watch out, because something was wrong with the way my mother treated me. I didn't understand where the voice was coming from; there was no one there. I also didn't recognize the voice, nor did I understand to what it was referring. My mother wasn't angry or upset with me at that moment. But the voice had sounded so clear and insistent, it jolted me into questioning my relationship with my mother for the first time.

Like most children, I believed my family was normal because I didn't know anything different. It felt normal that my mother's rules, moods, and beliefs ruled our house because no one, not even my father and grandparents (my mother's parents), challenged her. No one questioned my mother's decisions, her name-calling, her physical violence, or her infamous ability to dish out silent treatment whenever anyone upset her. As the eldest child, I was expected to be obedient and set a good example for my four siblings. And as the elder daughter, I was supposed to step into my mother's shoes and walk a repeat of her life. I grew up watching her anxiously anticipating *her* mother's every need, and I knew from a young age that this was what my mother wanted me to do for her. It wasn't until I was in my thirties that I realized how unbending my mother was, and that she wasn't going to renegotiate the rules she had set out for our relationship.

It's fair to say that the voice I heard in the bike stands when I was sixteen increased the conflict between my mother and I because it made me question whether I was responsible for her happiness. It created a gap between her voice, which I had learned to believe in, and my own voice that was starting to speak to me in louder whispers. I began to feel angry about having to apologize when I hadn't done anything wrong. Over time, I started to challenge myself to not give into my fear about upsetting Mom and to resist apologizing as long as I could.

Once, when I was nineteen, I held out for five days against apologizing for some infraction I wasn't aware I'd committed. On that Monday, Mom suddenly became angry with me and withdrew into her usual stony, angry silence. On Friday morning, as I sat at the piano to do my daily practice and yelled at my sister because I thought she had misplaced the piano music I needed, Mom's silent anger erupted into violence. Mom stormed into the room and started hitting me around the head. Mom hitting us wasn't an unusual event, but this was a frenzied attack. I shielded my head with my hands and waited until she was finished. Somehow her physical outburst helped her get over her anger, and she started talking to me again. And I felt victorious because I hadn't apologized when I had nothing for which to apologize. Again, it wasn't until I was in my thirties that I realized how abusive my mother had been that Friday morning—and how abusive it was to make me responsible for her unhappiness.

During my twenties, my relationship with Mom yo-yoed between us holding onto our silence until her coldness, or a family event I wanted to attend and couldn't until I apologized, or my emotional need for her, grew too much, and I would apologize for anything and everything. And each time I apologized, I hoped my mother would be different. I'd fantasize that she would somehow start listening to me and recognize that I had feelings of my own that deserved to be heard. But sadly, she never changed. She refused to listen to me right up until she died, which I since learned to understand was a result of her emotional health issues and extreme emotional starvation.

My mother lived a hard life. Underneath her extreme need for control was a hurt, angry girl who hadn't been listened to enough, or loved enough, by her parents and husband. My mother's mother was a stoic, emotionally silent woman who made my mother responsible for her unmet needs. Her own father was a controlling, emotionally manipulative man who criticized her whenever she did something he didn't agree with. And my father was a typical man of her generation, steadfast in his role as provider and emotionally unavailable. I believe my mother's behavior was a result of having experienced too much emotional neglect from her parents and husband, too much violence during the years she was held prisoner, at ten years old, in a Japanese concentration camp during the Second World War, and an overwhelming level of sexism that had stopped her from feeling entitled to be heard. And as her daughter, I was supposed to make all this pain go away.

At twenty-six, I had another big awakening when my daughter was born. As I wrote in my first book, *The Silent Female Scream*, when "I heard the midwife say that I had a daughter, a chill ran through my body and a voice in my head said, *If I don't get my shit straight, this new girl isn't going to have a happy life.*"[1] Like that voice at sixteen, this voice woke me up to knowing I could no longer delay in finding out what had gone wrong between my mother and I.

There was something different about having a daughter, rather than my son, who'd been born three years earlier. With Olivia, the legacy of unmothered daughters and emotionally neglected and invisible women that stretched far behind me felt dangerously close to infecting her life. I didn't want her to grow up feeling unmothered, invisible, and worried that her voice and feelings didn't matter. I didn't want her to come home every day from school with an anxious knot in her stomach, as I had, because she was worried I would be in a bad mood. I wanted her to grow up knowing that she was entitled to have her thoughts, feelings, and needs heard. I wanted her to grow up feeling free to be herself, and not be limited by the role expectations, myths, and stereotypes that had restricted my own and my mother's lives. I did not want her to inherit my family's generational belief that "good mothers and daughters" are selfless, self-denying, and self-sacrificing, because I had already learned from having watched my mother and grandmother that these role expectations are toxic to women's emotional wellbeing and mother-daughter relationships.

But knowing that something had to change is not the same as knowing how to change it. At twenty-six I had no role model who showed me how to mother differently. And in New Zealand during the 1980s there were no workshops or courses on the mother-daughter relationship or therapists who specialized in the mother-daughter relationship. So I devoured all the books I could find on women's rights and empowerment, including classics like *My Mother/My Self* by Nancy Friday, *The Cinderella Complex* by Colette Dowling, and *When You and Your Mother Can't Be Friends* by Victoria Secunda. I watched *The Oprah Winfrey Show* because she was the first woman I heard who spoke out about women's entitlement to speak their emotional truths. I talked to anyone and everyone about their mother-daughter relationship. And the more women I talked to, the more I realized that my mother and I weren't alone with our problems. I poured my heart out in my journals. And I went back to college to finish my Bachelor of Education degree at the University of Canterbury in Christchurch, even though it wasn't welcomed by my family or my in-law family.

I also created a parenting style where I put my children's needs first. At the time, I thought this was the answer to changing the generational pattern of unheard and unloved daughters. Putting my children's needs first was also the message of good mothering I was surrounded by. Since then, through my mother-daughter relationship research, and other scholarly research, I've learned that this parenting style only served to repeat in my life the selflessness, self-denial, and sacrifice that had harmed my mother's and grandmother's emotional wellbeing, limited their opportunities, and created a sticky, codependent relationship with each other. By denying my own needs I was showing my daughter that, as a girl, her needs mattered, but when she grew up and became a mother, her needs would evaporate because it would be her job to meet her children's, husband's, and family's needs.

After multiple moments of extreme exhaustion I finally woke up to how I had recreated my inherited pattern of self-neglect in nearly every part of my life. I had recreated it in my marriage and friendships because I rarely asked for help or support. I had recreated it in the way I mothered because I had made myself invisible as a person, and like my mother, I was setting my daughter up to meet my unvoiced needs. And I had recreated it in the way I squeezed my work around the edges of my family because I didn't believe I had the right to ask my family to make space for my work life.

What started as a personal quest quickly grew into my life's calling as I realized that my mother's and my conflict, though extreme, wasn't unusual. Despite the research on women's development, there is a worldwide epidemic of mother-daughter conflict that is screaming to be told, because solving the mother-daughter puzzle is essential for women's emotional development, emotional empowerment, and equality. Too many mothers and daughters are suffering from not feeling heard or understood, because the women's movement and counseling training courses largely ignore this key female relationship. And too many mothers and daughters feel ashamed of their conflict because they have been led to believe that their conflict is due to their own pathology, which in most cases is simply not true. Research clearly shows that mother-daughter conflict is a reflection of how women are treated in their generational family, culture, and society.

In 1993 I facilitated my first, and New Zealand's first, mother-daughter workshop, in the hall of St. Mark's Methodist Church in my hometown of Christchurch. This was a huge deal for me because back then I was terrified of public speaking. But as I discussed the mother-daughter relationship with about thirty women, I knew this was what I was going to do for the rest of my life. So when my husband and I and our two young children moved to Bloomington, Indiana in 1993, I applied and was admitted into the Counseling master's program at Indiana University.

Mom didn't cope well with my move to America. With too much generational trauma of loss and separation, and no voice to process her feelings, she returned every letter I wrote unopened, until she finally wrote to me, accusing me of being a bad daughter and asking me to stop writing because she no longer wanted to see me.

Reading her message, I had another moment where a voice saved me. As I sat on the bed tearfully looking at her hateful words, I suddenly felt a warm blanket being put around my shoulders and a voice saying, "Leave it to me, it's going to be all right."

The voice was correct. Without knowing it, or meaning to, my mother gave me my career. Thanks to her I have had the privilege of helping thousands of women over the years solve their mother-daughter puzzle and change harmful generational patterns and cultural beliefs.

After my graduation in 1997, our family moved to Nottingham, England, where I set up my private practice specializing in the mother-daughter relationship, which as far as I know is the first in the world. In 2011, my husband and I relocated to New Hampshire in the United States, where we live today.

I am blessed to have worked with so many courageous women and girls who have helped me uncover the mysteries of the mother-daughter relationship. And I am grateful to my fellow pioneers—you know who you are—who have invited me to give the keynote address at your conference, facilitate a workshop, or give a lecture, so I could disseminate my knowledge. But being a pioneer is hard, especially when the mother-daughter relationship is a marginalized subject in the counseling and coaching professions. Even though the counseling, social work, and coaching professions are female dominated, women have a hard time getting heard. The theories therapists use are often created by men, and the theories created by women are frequently ignored. And in many instances men, not women, are viewed as leaders. This has made it hard for me to be heard, especially since I talk about a female-only subject that holds patriarchy accountable for the damage it inflicts on mothers and daughters by the way it silences women's feelings, thoughts, and needs.[2]

Ironically, regardless of the wealth of research from feminist writers and academics, the women's movement has been just as culpable in the way it has ignored the power the mother-daughter relationship has to challenge sexist thinking and create gender equality. In their rush to enshrine gender equality into law, the women's movement has forgotten to address how women internalize the sexism they experience and how a daughter inherits her mother's internalized sexism.

I don't know why the women's movement has been reticent in engaging in this conversation and using it to change women's lives and relationships. It might be because they're afraid of being criticized for victim blaming, which is entirely unfounded. Understanding the way women internalize the sexism to which they're exposed is not victim blaming, it's emotionally empowering. Or is it because the women's movement has internalized the sexism that marginalizes the mother-daughter relationship into self-contained dyads, with separate issues such as mothers with "difficult" teenage daughters and adult daughters with "demanding" elderly mothers? As I show throughout this book, the mother-daughter relationship is a lifelong, three-generation relationship that tells the story of women's lives and how families, societies, cultures, and religions emotionally treat women.

Thankfully, as with all new ideas, there is a tipping point when suddenly a new idea becomes mainstream, and I am seeing this happen with the mother-daughter relationship. I am hearing more women and girls talking about how they recognize the importance of understanding their mother-daughter history and the themes and co-opted sexism being passed down the generations. Women and girls are talking about how the next stage of the women's movement involves claiming their entitlement to have their feelings and emotional needs inquired after and honored. Laws alone will not make women heard, or equal, as the Equal Pay Act of 1963 in the United States shows. It's time that women themselves speak out about what they need emotionally after generations of emotional silence and emotional neglect, because this conversation is essential for women's visibility and equality.

In this book I solve the mother-daughter puzzle by first laying out the puzzle pieces in Chapters 1 to 3. In Chapters 4 through 6, I put the puzzle together and describe in detail the three solutions in the *Mother-Daughter Coaching Model*™. In the final three chapters, I use the finished puzzle to heal and empower mothers and daughters. Empowering you, as the reader, as a mother or daughter, means teaching you how to voice what you feel, think, and emotionally need. Empowering you means learning how to speak and be heard, and learning how to listen to yourself and your mother or daughter. And it means knowing how to stand in each other's shoes so you understand each other's perspective.

Mother-Daughter History Mapping™ is the main learning exercise of the *Mother-Daughter Coaching Model.* In Chapter 6, I provide step-by-step instructions on how to map your mother-daughter history. The instructions are easy to follow and I encourage you to get together with a trusted friend, your mother, or your sister, and map each other's mother-daughter history through the telling of your stories and the excavation of the emotional reality the women in your generational family live. When you have completed the exercise, you will have a road map that outlines any harmful generational themes that need to be changed. And in Chapters 7 and 8, I teach you how to go about changing these destructive generational themes and beliefs.

Throughout *The Mother-Daughter Puzzle* I explain the mother-daughter relationship by telling some of my clients' mother-daughter stories. Because my clients' stories are confidential, I have changed all identifying names and details to preserve their anonymity, but you will certainly see yourself reflected in their stories. You will be able to empathize with Hannah and Ruth as they struggle to listen to each other and find a new way of relating for Hannah's new baby girl. You will cry as you read Sandeep's story, and you will understand how Katherine and Abigail feel. All these women tell the universal story of women's multigenerational experience with sexism, and how it harms the mother-daughter relationship. And I hope that this book will motivate you to join with other women and create your own *Women's Power Circle*™, where you support each other as you learn how to speak your emotional truth, raise your entitlement to be heard and emotionally supported, and change harmful generational beliefs and cultural patterns.

This book will empower mothers and daughters of all ages to understand each other and build relationships in which they feel heard, understood, emotionally supported, and loved. It will stop mothers from being fearful about their daughters turning thirteen, because they will understand that mother-daughter conflict when the daughter is an adolescent is not a foregone conclusion. It will stop mothers and daughters from feeling guilty about not being enough, or not doing enough. And it will inspire women to gather in circles and together create a world where women's emotional truth is valued, where women are allowed to be powerful on their terms.

Wishing you a strong voice, an emotionally connected relationship with your mother, or daughter, and a circle of empowered women around you!

With love,

Rosjke

PART ONE

LAYING OUT THE PUZZLE PIECES

CHAPTER 1

RUTH AND HANNAH

Different personality types and fluctuating hormones do not explain mother-daughter conflict.

LIKE MANY MOTHERS and daughters I work with, Ruth and Hannah were confused about what was causing them to argue over the smallest of things and resort to long periods of silence. Their friends and family members had told them that their relationship problems were a symptom of their differing personality types. Ruth, the mother, was a tall, elegantly dressed woman of fifty-five, with a beautifully coiffed gray bob, who sat perfectly upright in her chair in front of the computer as I worked with this mother-daughter couple through Skype. During the first session, she wore a stunning tailored blue jacket with white piping. Hannah, her daughter, looked quite different. At thirty-one, and heavily pregnant, her wild, curly blond hair hung loose around her shoulders, and during the first session she wore a white tee shirt under dungarees. At first meeting, I could see how emotionally different they were as well. Ruth was quiet and reserved and Hannah loud and talkative.

Ruth and Hannah had seen a therapist before they saw me, who had diagnosed their relationship problems as stemming from Ruth's passive-aggressive behavior. During our first session, I could see why the therapist had offered this diagnosis. The way Ruth dismissed Hannah's feelings did feel passive-aggressive. Yet as we dug below the surface of their relationship and understood how the women in their generational family were treated emotionally, we discovered that their different personality types and Ruth's passive-aggressive behavior weren't the root causes of their habitual arguments. As with all mothers and daughters, Ruth and Hannah's conflicted relationship and Ruth's passive-aggressive behavior are symptoms of a much bigger story—the story of how women are treated and have been treated over the generations.

Women's generational experience with sexism and gender inequality is the root cause of why mothers and daughters fight, misunderstand each other, and emotionally disconnect. In every mother-daughter relationship I work with, I see how mothers and daughters are set up for conflict. The background from which their struggle emerges are the ways mothers are expected to be selfless caretakers, the silencing of women's voices and emotional needs, and restrictive gender roles that limit women's choices and freedom. When women's voices are silenced by their family, culture, and wider society, mothers and daughters end up fighting over who gets to be heard. When women's emotional needs are not being inquired after, or met, mothers and daughters fight over whose needs get to be met in their relationship. When a mother's life is defined by her caregiving role, and her family provides little time or care for her as a person, the exhaustion and emotional neglect she feels will influence how she relates to her daughter, and her daughter can unconsciously inherit her mother's tendency to self-neglect.

As with all mothers and daughters, Ruth and Hannah's relationship was a window into what it was like to be female in their family. The way they argued told the story of what Ruth's life was like and what Ruth's mother's life was like, and of the emotional disempowerment and sexism being passed down from Ruth's mother to Ruth, and from Ruth to Hannah.

It was no surprise that Hannah initiated the decision to make an appointment with me, being the more vocal one in the relationship. But her assertiveness wasn't the only reason why she reached out for help. Being seven months' pregnant with her first child, a baby girl, made her miss her mom even more. She yearned to restore the emotional closeness she remembered having with her mom when she was a young girl, and she wanted her daughter to grow up surrounded by a loving mother-grandmother team, rather than a bickering, angry, hurting one.

As you'll learn about in Chapter 4, the mother-daughter relationship has distinct developmental stages, where the relationship comes under greater scrutiny and unresolved issues bubble up to the surface in hope of resolution. A daughter being pregnant and becoming a mother is one of these stages. Relationship cracks that have been ignored or papered over in the past make their presence felt, giving a mother and her daughter an opportunity to challenge and change what isn't working in their relationship.

This revealing of schisms and the desire to bridge them is especially true if a new baby daughter is on her way to join the mother-daughter team. The arrival of a new baby girl shines a spotlight on the experience of being female. Beliefs about femininity and motherhood are placed under the microscope. The mother, in this case Ruth, reminisces over what it was like for her when she was a young mother, and the pregnant daughter, Hannah, scrutinizes her mother's parenting style and life choices, and their relationship.

All this examination is good! If handled well, it can lead to profound change. Self-reflection increases a daughter's understanding about her mother's life, generating greater empathy and appreciation. Also, it provides both mother and daughter with powerful information on how to change destructive generational themes and sexist role-expectations. But when a mother and daughter are struggling to listen to each other and resolve painful issues, this kind of scrutiny puts an unbearable strain on an already fragile relationship.

By the time they came to see me, Ruth and Hannah's relationship was extremely fragile. Their relationship conflict started during Hannah's adolescence, which is common for mothers and daughters as a daughter is testing limits in preparation for adulthood. For some mothers and daughters, this adolescent conflict ends when the daughter reaches adulthood. But for Ruth and Hannah, the arguing and silent treatment that set the tone of Hannah's adolescence hadn't gone away. Now that Hannah was pregnant, she wanted to understand why she and her mother couldn't relate in a calm and loving way. Now that she and Ruth were at the next developmental stage of their relationship, the issues that had caused conflict when Hannah was an adolescent were screaming to be resolved.

Hannah was thankfully a wise mother-to-be. She instinctively knew that her relationship with her mother would influence how she and her daughter were going to relate, and she was terrified that her daughter would grow up feeling angry toward her, just as she had grown up feeling anger toward Ruth. During our first session Hannah said, "I want to change how Mom and I communicate, because this arguing isn't good for me, or my baby girl, and right now I really need Mom's love and support."

Ruth also felt hurt by the lack of connection she had with her only daughter. Hannah's growing animosity worried her, and she was tired of watching what she said to Hannah to avoid upsetting her. Ruth didn't want to lose her daughter and granddaughter, and knew this was a distinct possibility if their relationship didn't change. During our first session, Ruth said, "I often feel jealous when I see mothers and daughters out shopping together or having coffee. They all seem to be having such a good time, and I want the same for Hannah and me."

As Ruth and Hannah's therapy began, it was disturbing to see how angry they were with each other. I frequently had to stop them arguing because the smallest issue would set them yelling at each other. Their arguments would typically start with Hannah taking offense at something Ruth had said, and Ruth reacting in a defensive manner because she didn't understand what she had done wrong. And then the loud arguing would start. Neither of them knew how to listen to each other's feelings and needs. And because mothers and daughters are like elephants that never forget their past, especially past hurt, every unresolved argument added another painful justification in Ruth and Hannah's minds about why they weren't destined to have an emotionally close relationship.

On one occasion, Ruth asked me if I thought Hannah's pregnancy hormones were to blame for Hannah's behavior. Hannah exploded at this suggestion, and while I calmed her down, I explained that Hannah's hormones weren't to blame. In my view, hormones or hormone imbalances don't cause mother-daughter conflict. Blaming women's hormones is a common sexist strategy that is designed to dismiss women's truth and protect perpetrators from being accountable for their abusive behavior. This strategy also protects patriarchal (male-controlled or male-dominant) societies from being made to acknowledge how they deliberately undervalue and neglect women's rights, and the emotional harm this inflicts on women.

Even though Ruth's question about pregnancy hormones triggered intense anger in Hannah, I felt this theme deserved closer scrutiny because it provided an important clue as to what it was like to be female in their family. If Ruth thought that her daughter's ire was connected to her pregnancy hormones, chances were Ruth herself had learned to brush aside her own feelings as hormonal, and therefore irrelevant, rather than a warning sign that something was wrong or that something important was missing for her.

When I asked Ruth why she thought Hannah's hormones might be to blame, Ruth explained that she wasn't trying to discount Hannah's feelings or absolve herself from being responsible for upsetting Hannah. She said she asked this question because her husband and mother, Hannah's grandmother, often accused her of being "hormonal." In this generational family, women had no voice. Whenever they cried out in protest or complained about how they were being treated, their feelings were attributed to them being hormonal.

Understanding Ruth and Hannah's Generational History

It was time to map Ruth's mother-daughter history. Mapping a woman's mother-daughter history is an insightful diagnostic tool I developed that reveals the truth about women's generational experience with sexism and gender inequality. It maps out the stories of my client's, her mother's, and her grandmother's lives, including whether these women's voices were silenced or heard, their emotional needs dismissed or facilitated, and how the sexism in their generation limited their choices and opportunities. Through the mapping of a woman's mother-daughter history, answers are found as to why she is struggling with certain emotional or mental issues, why her relationship with her mother or daughter is troubled, and what themes and self-defeating beliefs she inherited from her mother.

As we mapped Ruth's mother-daughter history, it didn't take long for the theme of emotional neglect to be uncovered. Behind the façade of wealth and comfort in which Ruth, her mother, and her grandmother had lived, lay the more important reality of how these three women were emotionally neglected by their husbands, parents, and other family members. Even though Ruth lived in a beautiful home, drove an expensive foreign car, and wore fashionable clothes that her friends envied, Ruth was an emotionally starved woman whose worth and life were defined by her being a dutiful wife and mother. Ruth's husband treated his wife as if she was in service to him and his work, and Ruth's mother never inquired after how Ruth was feeling or whether she was happy. Hannah was the only person who asked her what she wanted, which caused a great deal of conflict in their relationship, because Ruth didn't know how to answer her daughter. I had a hunch that the reason Ruth resorted to being silent, or why she criticized her daughter for some unrelated issue, was because she felt uncomfortable about not knowing how to voice her thoughts and feelings.

Ruth and her mother had married successful businessmen who were married more to their work than their wives. Both lived a sort of "Stepford Wives" existence in which they maintained perfectly appointed houses and well-groomed bodies. Ruth had learned from her mother how to be a charming host for her husband's frequent business dinners, even when she wasn't feeling well. And she had learned to tolerate being alone most evenings and weekends while her husband had business engagements.

As Ruth looked at her completed mother-daughter history map, she recognized for the first time how neglected she was. She told Hannah and me the story of how she had wanted to call off her wedding weeks before the wedding day because she was worried about how preoccupied

Frank, her husband-to-be, was about his work. But her mother had persuaded her to go ahead and marry Frank. Ruth said her mother told her she was extremely lucky to have secured "such a fine catch."

Ruth took a deep breath and said in a barely audible whisper, "Mom made me believe that I couldn't ask Frank to spend more time with me because successful men have to put all their energy into their work. She made me believe I wasn't important, and that I was lucky to be marrying Frank because everyone was jealous of me. She never said that Frank was lucky to be marrying me. And now this map is making me feel angry at Mom for not listening to my doubts about marrying Frank. Why didn't my happiness matter to her?"

Ruth's words echoed around the room, and I saw Hannah soften toward her mother. As it turned out, this was the first time Hannah had heard this story. She knew that her father was neglectful of her mother, but she had always blamed her mother for it. She was angry with her mother for putting up with her father's neglect. But, after hearing how invisible her mother had been when she was a young woman, and how invisible her grandmother had been, and that no one in Ruth's life cared about what Ruth thought and felt, she realized it wasn't right or fair to blame her mother for her father's neglectful behavior.

I agreed with Hannah. It wasn't fair to blame Ruth for how her husband treated her, and it wasn't fair to blame Ruth's mother for teaching her daughter to tolerate an abusive marriage. Neither woman knew that something different was possible. No one had ever asked Ruth's mother what she needed, or what made her happy. Ruth's mother didn't know how to ask her daughter these important questions.

Blaming Frank for how he neglected Ruth and Hannah doesn't tell the full story either. Frank will always be responsible for his abusive neglect, but his behavior also needs to be understood within a wider generational context, where he learned from his father, and his father from his grandfather, how to emotionally neglect women, and to believe that the only mark of a successful man was to be financially successful and a good provider.

Seeing the strong theme of emotional neglect and emotional starvation in her mother's mother-daughter history map gave Hannah the words to describe what she believed was causing their conflict. Hannah didn't want to step into her mother's shoes and repeat her mother's emotionally unsupported life. She didn't want to dedicate her life to her husband's career or her family's needs. She didn't want to spend hours alone while her husband worked or traveled abroad. And she felt that Ruth didn't understand this. To me Hannah said, "Mom doesn't know how to relate to me because my life is so very different from hers."

Changing Generational Themes

Thus, Hannah became a pioneer for change in her generational family. She saw the damage that her family's definition of motherhood had inflicted on her mother, and grandmother, and she was desperate to live by a new standard. She had also chosen to marry a different kind of man from her father. Hannah's husband was an enlightened man who was willing to be an equal partner and hands-on parent. He, too, witnessed the suffering his mother and grandmother had endured from their emotionally neglectful husbands, and he didn't want to treat his wife that way.

While we talked about the generational theme of emotional neglect, Ruth said something she hadn't said before: "Of late I've been feeling increasingly frustrated with my life. I'm tired of being alone at night. I'm tired of being at Frank's, and everyone else's, beck and call. And I'm exhausted from being shown off whenever Frank wants me to be. I never realized how much I've repeated my mother's life until now." And having said this, Ruth turned to Hannah and said, "I would love to have your help in changing all of this."

Changing this inherited theme became the goal of their therapy, and with my guidance Ruth learned how to start to listen to herself, and Ruth and Hannah to listen to each other. On one occasion, Ruth was able to hear and respond to Hannah's anger about how her doctor had dismissed her during one of her prenatal visits. In the past, Ruth would have discounted Hannah's feelings with some vague comment, which would have sparked an argument. But this time Ruth empathized with Hannah, and helped her process what she was going to do about it. This was a moment of celebration!

Ruth also learned to peel herself away from the corporate-wife role she had inhabited all her adult life, and started discovering who she was and what she wanted. I coached her on how to practice the simple but difficult exercise of waking up her inner voice that let her know what she was feeling and wanting. I encouraged her to disregard the guilt she had learned to feel when she said no to someone, because this kind of guilt isn't true guilt. It is guilt by proxy, which I explain in Chapter 8. And I instructed her about how a real friendship feels and behaves, because Ruth's idea of a good relationship meant being invisible.

The stronger Ruth grew emotionally, the more her life changed. She sold her expensive foreign car and bought a car she liked more, though her husband was furious with her for doing this. She changed the way she dressed, which is often a sign that things are changing for the better. And Ruth's friendship group changed to include caring and empowering women.

Even though Hannah was more in tune with her inner voice than Ruth, she, too, had inherited some of her mother's emotional silencing, which she challenged and changed. She also became aware of how she misdirected the anger she felt toward her father to her mother. Like many daughters of neglectful fathers, she directed the hurt she felt about her father's disinterest in her to her mother, because Ruth was the safest and most available parent to feel angry with. As we talked about this dynamic, Ruth shared how she felt responsible to make up for what Frank didn't provide for his children. For homework, I instructed Ruth and Hannah to create a ceremony together, without Frank, where they had to return the responsibility Frank had to both listen to, and emotionally support, his wife and daughter, back to him, regardless of whether he recognized this responsibility or not. They created a wonderful ceremony where they wrote poems and read them out to each other, and then burned them in a fire pit to release their words back to the universe.

Ruth and Hannah have a very bright future ahead of them. These two women, along with Hannah's husband, are pioneering a new family environment where women's emotional needs are voiced. Their story shows the power the mother-daughter relationship has to change harmful beliefs and practices for future generations. Sadly, Ruth's husband chose to be angry about the changes Ruth and Hannah were making. In Frank's mind, his rules were perfectly reasonable and he wasn't going to change them. I don't know if Ruth's marriage survived, but I doubt it. Ruth's personal growth wouldn't have tolerated remaining in a marriage where she wasn't lovingly supported.

CHAPTER 2

THE LINK BETWEEN MOTHER-DAUGHTER CONFLICT AND SEXISM

When women are silenced, mothers and daughters learn to silence each other.

I HAVE HAD THE privilege of listening to thousands of mothers and daughters, mothers and daughters-in-law, and stepmothers and daughters talking about their relationship. Since the advent of Skype and online therapy, I've been able to work with mothers and daughters from around the world. This breadth of experience has taught me that unraveling the complicated dynamics between mothers and daughters and healing today's epidemic in mother-daughter conflict requires an exploration of women's multigenerational experience with sexism and gender inequality.

It makes sense that sexist beliefs and restrictive gender-role stereotypes that shape women's lives will have a detrimental impact on how mothers and daughters relate. We need to understand how the dramatic changes in women's lives over the past generations, which have increased opportunities and freedoms for daughters, are contributing to today's epidemic of mother-daughter conflict. We need to dig below the surface and uncover how women's multigenerational experience with emotional silence and emotional neglect harms a mother and daughter's ability to listen to themselves and each other. And we need to expose how the marginalization and depreciation of the mother-daughter relationship against the mother-son relationship and father-daughter relationship harms a mother and daughter's ability to value their rights and worth as women. In this chapter, I describe how the changes in women's roles, women's multigenerational experience with sexism, and the continued marginalization of the mother-daughter relationship, are the underlying factors that cause mothers and daughters around the world to fight and emotionally disconnect.

Changes in Women's Roles

In previous generations, when women's roles were more static, the mother-daughter relationship was defined by a strong symmetry or sameness. Typically, a daughter would step into her mother's shoes and perform the same roles and tasks her mother performed. And they would share the same beliefs about what it means to be female. But over the last two generations, this symmetry has been eroded. As women gained greater access to educational opportunities and professions, prospects from which their mothers were barred, daughters no longer stepped into their mother's shoes and walked a repeat of their mother's life. This means that mothers and daughters today have to find a way to connect from a place of difference. They have to find a way to talk about, and accept, their divergent opportunities, experiences, views, and definitions of femininity and motherhood.

For some mothers and daughters, being different isn't a problem. They eagerly revise their beliefs and incorporate their new roles and opportunities into their relationship. For these mothers and daughters, life is a journey of change and discovery. For others, change doesn't happen without a fight. For these mothers and daughters, being different feels like a personal attack, a rejection of the values they hold dear as they fight over who is right and who is wrong.

The most common side effect of the changes in women's roles I see between mothers and daughters is the mother feeling secretly jealous of her daughter's increased opportunities, choices, and freedoms. This issue is a difficult one to detect. I rarely hear a mother admit to being jealous of her daughter, because she was told by society these feelings of jealousy are wrong and shameful. I also find that most mothers are unaware they're feeling jealous of their daughter. They hide it away beneath being critical of their daughter's beliefs, behaviors, and choices, or by being emotionally unavailable.

Daughters too can find it hard to detect when their mother is jealous of them. Their mother's emotional withdrawal or criticisms can feel confusing, hurtful, and unwarranted. And because daughters are emotionally wired to make their mother happy, a daughter can internalize her mother's hurtful behavior by blaming herself for somehow causing her mother's unhappiness.

I have worked with many adolescent and adult daughters who were struggling with a cold, critical, and emotionally distant mother. For example, one daughter was hurt about her mother's lack of excitement when she won a much-coveted promotion at work. Another daughter was confused as to why her mother kept criticizing her kind and loving boyfriend. Another daughter was upset about how her mother was trying to sabotage her wedding day.

Unraveling what's going on in these and many other situations like them involves uncovering the role maternal jealousy might be playing in their relationship. It means exploring how a mother's jealousy of her daughter's life might be lurking as an unseen and unspoken reason for a mother's abusive and hurtful behavior. Discovering the root causes also means not blaming mothers for being jealous of their daughters. Society, and sadly the counseling and psychotherapy community, are quick to diagnose mothers as being the problem and blame them for harming their daughters. Yes, it is important to acknowledge that picking at your daughter's self-worth and being emotionally unavailable are abusive behaviors. But if we stop here and don't look deeper at what's causing a mother to be overly critical or emotionally withdrawn, maternal jealousy will never be fully understood; mothers will continue to be unfairly blamed, and mothers and daughters will never really understand each other.

At its heart, maternal jealousy tells the story of the grief mothers feel when they realize, through their daughters' lives, what they missed out on in their own lives. When we look back at the restrictions our mothers had to endure, and the dreams and potential they never got to realize, jealousy of today's opportunities and freedoms makes sense. Generations ago, when mothers and daughters lived the same restricted life, mothers were unaware that more was possible. But daughters today are showing their mothers the opportunities they didn't get to have, the love they didn't receive, and the freedom they didn't get to enjoy. This is an exceedingly painful truth for mothers to face! And their pain is made worse when mothers are blamed for feeling these normal human emotions.

Mothers and daughters both bear the brunt of the sexism that patriarchy has inflicted on generations of women. And when families don't talk about the quite normal grief mothers feel about what they never got to be and do, a daughter is in danger of becoming an increasingly uncomfortable mirror for her mother. This silence can result in mothers and daughters being unaware of what's hindering their ability to feel close to each other. The daughter becomes a too-painful reminder of what her mother wanted, but never got to have, and for some mothers, this pain is unbearable. Their unvoiced and shame-filled pain can make it too hard for them to be emotionally supportive of their daughter and enjoy the closeness their daughter desires.

My work with daughters who are struggling with their mother's jealousy involves helping them understand their mother's life more closely and recognize the real reasons for their mother's hurtful behavior. I show them that their mother's upsetting behavior is coming from the mother's life experiences and the sexism that limited her options. And I help them understand that even though it feels personal, at some level it isn't. Their mother is misdirecting the anger and resentment she feels about how her patriarchal family and society mistreated her toward her daughter, because her daughter is the closest person to her.

In my work with the abovementioned daughters, one daughter discovered that her grandfather had stopped her mother from going to college. The daughter's college degree and her recent promotion at work were hard for her mother to celebrate, because they were reminders of what she wanted but never had the chance to have. Another daughter learned to see with new eyes how unloving and emotionally abusive her father was toward her mother, and how her loving, supportive boyfriend was a painful mirror for her mother to look at and see the neglect and lack of love she had learned to tolerate from her husband. The third daughter learned that her mother was sabotaging her wedding day because her mother's family had made her marry in secret because she was pregnant. The daughter's wedding preparations and dress-fitting sessions were reminders of her mother's own shame-filled wedding day, and how she never got to wear a beautiful dress or be celebrated.

By putting a factual context around their mother's hurtful behavior, I was able to help these daughters increase the empathy they felt for their mother, and clear up any worry they felt that they were somehow responsible for their mother's unhappiness. My research shows that this kind of historical exploration sets daughters free to claim their dreams and opportunities, helping them to avoid repeating the restrictions and sacrifices under which their mothers suffered. And it teaches daughters to love the mother they have and not inherit their mother's unhappiness or tolerate their mother's abusive behavior.

Mothers and daughters owe it to themselves to dig below their emotionally distant or hurtful behavior and understand what life experiences have made them behave in this way. This kind of emotional excavation teaches women about their female history. It tells a daughter the stories of her mother's life and provides the healing balm of being known, even if some mothers find it too painful to tell their story. It stops daughters from internalizing their mother's grief and blaming themselves for having made their mother unhappy. It stops daughters from stepping into their mother's shoes and repeating the restrictions in their mother's life. And it passes back the blame for our mother's pain about her lost dreams and unrealized potential to the culture and society that shamefully and selfishly put her in service to her husband and family, rather than giving her the dignity she deserved to be free to be herself.

Tragically, maternal jealousy poisoned my relationship with my mother. My mother should have had more opportunities than she did. And then because this conversation wasn't spoken in my family, my success as our family's first woman to receive a bachelor's and master's degree was never celebrated.

In my family, daughters are expected to step into their mother's shoes and walk a repeat of their mother's life as a mark of respect for our mother. My grandmother stepped into her mother's shoes, and my mother stepped into my grandmother's shoes, and I was expected to step into my mother's shoes. Our relationship troubles started when I refused to step into my mother's shoes.

For years I thought that my mother's soul-cutting criticism, the way she would lash out in anger for no apparent reason, and her annual excuse to ignore my birthday, was my fault. I thought I had caused my mother to behave like this, until I dug below the surface and recognized her anger wasn't about me, though it was directed at me. I realized that Mom's anger was because I was a living reminder of all she did not get to be and do. When I uncovered this deeper truth, I knew I wasn't the cause of my mother's hurt and that I wasn't responsible for her anger. And for my own and my daughter's sake, I shouldn't shrink down to spare my mom from feeling her pain. I realized I must live and dream, and take hold of every opportunity, because if I didn't, history would repeat itself and my daughter would end up being the object of my jealousy.

Imagine, for a moment, if the resentment women feel about the limitations they have had to live with was given a voice. I don't think we know the half of what would come bursting forth from the depths of women's hearts. Imagine the power these voices would have to stop women from feeling guilty about the sexist and abusive ways they've been treated. When women tell their stories and we hear the secrets they carry about how men have mistreated them, how religions have blamed and shamed them, and how patriarchy has controlled women's bodies, autonomy, and rights, our world is changed forever.

The Multigenerational Impact of Sexism

Lily Myers's YouTube poem *Shrinking Women* is an accurate and astute account of the emotional impact of women's multigenerational history with sexism.[1] Lily talks about how she denies herself the food she wants, just like her mother does. How she overaccommodates other people's needs and underaccommodates her own, just like her mother does. How she apologizes for speaking her truth because she feels responsible for upsetting people, just like her mother does. And that she feels uncomfortable with taking up all the physical space she needs, just like her mother does. I'm not surprised this poem went viral. It speaks of the female experience of how sexism teaches women to underaccommodate themselves, to filter their voices, to deprive themselves of food and comfort, to make space for people who do not make space for them, and how these themes are passed on from mother to daughter.

When Katherine heard Lily's poem, she felt as if it had been written for her. Katherine knew how to shrink herself down in her relationships with men until there was little space left for her. And as she repeatedly listened to Lily's poem, she realized she didn't know how to claim space for herself. Nor did she know how to check whether a man was capable of making space for her, of loving her, and of being emotionally supportive. Lily's poem motivated Katherine to make an appointment with me, because she wanted to become aware of the unconscious emotional legacy she had inherited from her mother so she could change the disempowering beliefs and behaviors she was carrying around in her head.

When we mapped Katherine's mother-daughter history, we discovered how emotionally mute the women in her family were. Her mother and grandmother had learned to believe that "good women" should always honor and respect other people's feelings, even if it meant disrespecting and ignoring their own. And because they had learned to disregard their own feelings and needs, Katherine's mother and grandmother were classic martyrs, carrying their martyrdom as a badge of honor, and criticizing other women who didn't carry this badge as well.

When Katherine looked at her completed *Mother-Daughter History Map*, she saw how dangerous her mother's and grandmother's martyrdom was. She saw how it had disabled their ability to advocate for themselves. How it had made them vulnerable to being used and abused. How it had enabled her father and grandfather to bully their wives and feel an exaggerated sense of entitlement to be in charge. And she saw how this emotional legacy was linked to her tendency to tolerate unsupportive, controlling boyfriends.

At twenty-seven, Katherine had a history of dating selfish, overentitled, goal-focused men who expected her to be undemanding and focused on them. Her relationships would follow a predictable pattern of Katherine fitting in with what her boyfriend liked to do. But after some time of being superaccommodating, Katherine would start to feel unloved and irritated by her boyfriend's neglect. This would lead her to pick fights with her boyfriend in the hope that it would jolt him into showing her some care and attention. Predictably, the conflict would only lead to her boyfriend ending the relationship and calling her names like "crazy bitch."

During one of her sessions, Katherine admitted that she had never ended a relationship, including the one where her boyfriend had hit her. She had never told anyone that a previous boyfriend had hit her, because she felt ashamed about it. But when she connected the dots between how unentitled she felt to be heard, supported, and equal in her relationships, and how invisible her mother and grandmother had been next to their selfish and controlling husbands, her shame melted away. She realized that she had been set up by her generational legacy to be invisible in her relationships. That she was repeating the invisibility and disempowerment she had learned from her mother and grandmother. Knowing this energized her to start claiming her voice and space.

Katherine worked hard on changing her inherited legacy of martyred self-silencing and self-neglect. Sadly, this didn't have a positive effect on her relationship with her mother. For this mother and daughter, change didn't come without a fight. Katherine's mother couldn't let go of her martyrdom. She believed that Katherine's newfound assertiveness was not only unfeminine, but was also a rejection of their family's beliefs. Katherine's mother felt rejected by Katherine, who no longer wanted to join her mother in their conversations about how rude and uncaring people were. I also suspected that Katherine's mother was jealous of Katherine's newfound boldness and how loving Katherine's new boyfriend was. Katherine's life had become an uncomfortable mirror for her mother to look at, which her mother reacted against by being critical and emotionally withholding. This left Katherine with the difficult task of accepting that she didn't have the mother she needed while trying to love the one she had.

Marginalization of the Mother-Daughter Relationship

Even though women's issues are increasingly being addressed, the mother-daughter relationship remains one of the most disregarded topics within women's studies, psychotherapy, and feminism. With some notable exceptions, it is practically invisible in psychotherapy, counseling psychology, coaching, and social work training programs, women's studies programs, and women's conferences. For example, though my counseling training at Indiana University was first-class, it didn't include the mother-daughter relationship, even in the women's development course.

I find this omission inexcusable. It begs the question of how psychotherapy, coaching, and social work training courses can adequately prepare their graduates to understand women's lives and heal their emotional health issues without any consideration of what daughters inherit from their mothers. How can women's conferences and feminist conferences effectively empower women to claim their equal rights without a conversation about women's mother-daughter history, and how a mother's desire to make life better for her daughter fueled every right and freedom we now have? The birth of my daughter sparked my lifelong dedication to empowering mothers and daughters. Mothers' desire to make life better for their daughters energized visionary revolutionaries like Mary

Wollstonecraft, the suffragettes, and Jennifer Siebel Newsom, who created the documentary *Miss Representation*.[2] And how can business conferences empower women to shatter glass ceilings and claim their space in corporate boardrooms or as partners of law firms, for example, without a conversation about how sexism is internalized and passed on from mother to daughter?

Yet however frustrating this situation is, railing against it doesn't solve it. The solution to this problem requires a more sociological understanding of why it is in patriarchy's best interests to dismiss the mother-daughter relationship. Adrienne Rich alludes to this in her book *Of Women Born*, by explaining that the reason the mother-daughter relationship is "minimized and trivialized" by patriarchal institutions like academia, theology, sociology, art, and psychology, is because it is "profoundly threatening to men" and male domination.[3] Elizabeth Debold, Marie Wilson, and Idelisse Malave reiterate this in *Mother Daughter Revolution*, writing that the empowerment of the mother-daughter relationship involves "voice lessons that encourage resistance" to female inequality and male domination.[4] Additionally, each case study in this book confirms how much the mother-daughter relationship is a powerhouse for change and a threat to patriarchal beliefs and power.

When we recognize the power the mother-daughter relationship has to challenge and change sexist beliefs, harmful cultural practices, and discriminating religious doctrine, it makes sense that a patriarchal society will marginalize and trivialize the mother-daughter relationship. I see on a daily basis how mothers and daughters change the power imbalance in families and create family environments where females are respected as equals. I see how understanding the mother-daughter dynamic empowers women to claim their voice and create families and organizations that serve both women's and men's needs. And I see how understanding what we have inherited from our mothers empowers women to claim their voice and visibility in their relationships and reach their career potential.

When we delve into the often-confusing dynamics between mothers and daughters, something wonderful happens. Women learn about who they are. Women learn about why they believe what they believe and why they make the choices they make. Women learn about their female history, including how patriarchal thinking and sexist beliefs restricted their mother and grandmother's lives, limited their powers, and harmed their emotional wellbeing. We learn how women and families internalize these sexist beliefs and pass them on from mother to daughter. We see with clear-eyed clarity how, as Jack Holland writes in *Misogyny: The World's Oldest Prejudice*, the hatred of women and the desire to control women's bodies, minds, and lives forms the underlying motivation behind many political decisions, religious doctrines, and family decisions.[5]

In great part, *The Mother-Daughter Puzzle* is a call for religious leaders, helping professionals, and the women's movement to take a good, hard look at how they are perpetuating the marginalization of the mother-daughter relationship, and to examine how they devalue this vital female relationship and omit it from their courses and conferences. I hope that in the near future the mother-daughter relationship will be recognized for what it is: a hub of activism that emboldens women to challenge and change cultural practices and sexist thinking that harms women's bodies, minds, and rights.

The good news is, women already know how vitally important their relationship with their mother or daughter is. You see this power at work every time women gather. I guarantee that the next time you're with a group of women, within five minutes someone will share a story about their mother, grandmother, or daughter. And that someone will talk about how they wish their mother or daughter had more freedom, increased opportunities, and greater confidence to speak and be heard.

In the next chapter, I reveal the dark underbelly of the age-old role expectation that women should selflessly give of themselves. Selflessness, sacrifice, and service are at the heart of women's multigenerational experience with sexism, and they still express today's definition of femininity and motherhood. As the story of a young woman named Sandeep will show, these role expectations have disastrous consequences for women's emotional wellbeing, the mother-daughter relationship, and equality.

CHAPTER 3

HOW SELFLESS CAREGIVING HARMS THE MOTHER-DAUGHTER RELATIONSHIP

Caregiving is not just a female quality, it's a human quality.

AT A WOMEN'S business conference at Nottingham University in England, I attended a workshop on how to communicate with men. I was hoping to learn some tips for how I could communicate better with husbands and fathers about how they could support their wives and daughters. The workshop was presented by two enthusiastic men in their mid-twenties, who opened the workshop by informing us we should be aware that men are still wired like cavemen. They explained that in a man's caveman-like brain, he can struggle to hear a woman say "no," and instead hear "maybe," "possibly," and sometimes even "yes."

As I listened to this theory, my internal sexism detector started to scream loudly. The theory sounded so ridiculous, and so archaic, I couldn't believe they were being serious. I wondered if they were using it to make a joke, to jolt the audience into a reaction. But no one reacted. No one laughed, or spoke. And then it hit me: They weren't joking. They were deadly serious. These presenters actually believed this archaic, sexist theory that men aren't always able to hear a woman say no. And their goal for this workshop was to inform women of this so-called fact and instruct us on how we could make allowances for it in our interactions with men.

My hand shot up before my brain could stop me from speaking out. I asked the presenters how their theory would fit with a man not hearing a woman say no to his unwanted sexual advances. I asked if they were suggesting that in these situations women should make allowances for men not being able to hear them say no. Both men looked extremely uncomfortable with my question. Instead of giving me a direct answer, one spluttered an incoherent joke, and the other moved on to the next topic.

I was stunned. Who had invited these men to present? And did the conference organizers know what they were going to say? Hoping for some solidarity, I looked around the room for an ally but couldn't detect anyone feeling as uncomfortable as I was. I saw a room full of innovative women who were passively listening to this sexist message. Maybe inwardly someone else had reacted, but because she said nothing, her silence communicated her lack of objection. Knowing I wasn't going to be able to concentrate on the rest of the workshop, I got up and left.

Sadly, this was not an isolated incident of my witnessing women failing to challenge a sexist message. Something similar happened at a Springboard course I attended in 2000, while I was working as a counselor at Nottingham Trent University, England. Springboard is a women's empowerment program, facilitated in universities and organizations throughout England. During a discussion about the differences between being assertive and aggressive, the topic was raised about how women say no. The group of about twenty women believed that a woman is being aggressive if she says no without explaining why.

Again my internal sexism detector started to scream. I was reacting to the disparity between a man's no being taken as complete of itself, and a woman having to explain her no. But when I voiced this concern to the group, they united in counseling me to change my viewpoint. They suggested that if I didn't explain myself, people wouldn't like me because they would think I was an aggressive, self-centered woman. To be fair, they were correct in believing this. The university's organizational culture at that time didn't approve of assertive women. Women who advocated for what they wanted were often accused by the male hierarchy as lacking leadership qualities, as not team players, and as troublemakers. These accusations were successful in keeping women silent and away from positions of power.

In both of these examples, the women had internalized the sexism in their workplace to such a degree, they no longer recognized it as sexist. They had learned to believe in the sexist thinking that women, not men, have to explain themselves, that women are accommodating and self-sacrificing, and that women's feelings and needs don't matter that much. They had learned to know that surviving at work required that they played by these rules, somewhat like how captives can suffer from Stockholm syndrome, where they learn to overidentify with and oversympathize with their captors.

While the message is less overt today, it still exists. Why is this still happening after more than a century of feminist revolution? Why did those women not frog-march the two sexist presenters out of the building at the women's business conference? And why didn't the women at the Springboard course join together to challenge the sexism in their workplace?

Culture of Female Service

The answer to these questions lies in understanding our centuries-old belief in the "Culture of Female Service."[1] I coined this term because my clients needed an umbrella term that collects together all the ways society believes that it is a woman's God-given duty to be of service. And as the client stories in this book show, the Culture of Female Service is not limited to a particular culture or economic class. Even though women are gaining power and visibility in many countries around the world as prime ministers, presidents, and leaders of industry, emotionally we are still very much wedded to the belief that it is a woman's role to be of service. Motherhood, particularly, is still prone to being demarcated as a selfless, sacrificial role. From long before our grandmother's day, women's lives have been regarded as an all-consuming caregiving role that doesn't allow women an identity of their own. What women need hasn't had a voice, because historically women have been treated as listeners, rather than speakers, and care providers, rather than care receivers.

The truth is, this much-revered belief system has a dark underbelly. As the two experiences above show, it threatens women into cooperating with their own emotional silencing, emotional disempowerment, and inequality, by assigning negative connotations to women needing, women speaking up, and women being assertive. It sets mothers and daughters up to fight over their shared experience of being selfless. It sets women up to police each other's compliance with the rule that it is selfish to put your own needs before other people's needs. And these harmful beliefs are contagious. When daughters witness their father ignoring their mother's needs and their mother accepting this emotional neglect, they learn to comply with the Culture of Female Service's belief that women's needs don't exist. When a daughter sees her mother keeping quiet in order to keep the peace, the daughter learns to question the legitimacy of her truth, and her right to have her feelings and needs heard. When a daughter hears her mother agreeing to do something she hasn't got time for, the daughter learns that other people's needs are more important than her own. When a daughter hears her mother being praised for her selfless caregiving, she learns to feel ashamed of her desires and learns to connect self-neglect with being liked. And when women's wishes are challenged, daughters learn to want what other people want them to have, rather than what they want for themselves. While daughters are learning these lessons, they're often angry with their mothers for teaching them how to tolerate being unheard and invisible.

The above two incidents aren't just about women's lack of assertiveness. They are about the sexism women internalize from today's culture, and the sexism they have inherited from their mothers. If we don't look beyond the problem of women not knowing how to insist that their no is heard, no explanation necessary, we'll miss learning how the Culture of Female Service is still teaching women and girls today how to say yes when they want to say no, to listen rather than to speak, and to normalize how awful it feels to be the invisible caretaker in their relationships and at work.

Sandeep's Mother-Daughter Story

Sandeep's mother-daughter story reveals how dark the underbelly of the Culture of Female Service can get. Her story shows how women's emotional and mental wellbeing, equality and power, and mother-daughter relationships are damaged when families use their culture and religion to justify treating mothers and daughters as unpaid servants and wombs that birth much-desired sons.

When I met Sandeep, she was a twenty-two-year-old college student who lived at home with her parents and three brothers. Her Indian parents had immigrated to England before Sandeep was born. Sandeep's mother was in her late forties, and prone to bouts of illness. Her father was a respected businessman and community leader.

Sandeep came to see me because she was feeling depressed. She was struggling to complete her final year at the local university, along with doing all the shopping, cooking and cleaning for her family and caring for her frequently ill mother. She was angry that her parents expected her to do all the domestic work while her brothers were free to do whatever they wanted. She was also feeling conflicted between wanting to take care of her mom and feeling resentful about how ungrateful her mother was about all she did for her and her family.

"Mom criticizes everything I do," Sandeep told me. "Whatever I do isn't good enough, and she is making it harder for me to go to class. I do not know what to do because my mom needs me and I need to go to class."

The pressure to be an obedient, caring daughter weighed heavily on Sandeep. She loved her mom and she desperately wanted to take care of her and make her happy. She felt guilty that she wasn't doing enough for her mom, and labored under an additional guilt over not having enough time for her studies. Sandeep wanted to graduate, but her loyalty toward her mom, and her family's attitude that Sandeep's main purpose in life was to take care of her family, were making it difficult.

Sandeep's family was highly patriarchal. Fathers, husbands, and sons set the rules, and mothers, wives, and daughters obeyed them. Sandeep's mother and grandmother were each in an arranged marriage with an abusive, controlling husband who expected his wife to ask his permission for nearly everything. When Sandeep's aunt came for a visit from India, she told Sandeep how her grandmother used to take out the abuse she experienced from her husband on her daughter, Sandeep's mom. Sandeep's aunt told her stories of how her grandmother used to hit her mother when she was a young girl, and say to her that no decent man would ever want to marry her because she was a bad housekeeper. Sandeep's mother was taken out of school when she was only twelve years old, so she could devote all of her time to doing the housework, while her brothers finished school and some even graduated from university.

Sandeep cried as she told me these stories. She continued to tell me how years ago, her father had refused to give her mother permission to go to India to visit her dying brother. "Dad told everyone that he couldn't afford it, even though I know this wasn't true," she said between sniffles. "Dad had gone back to India regularly without my mom. No one challenged Dad's decision, or stood up for my mom. Everyone acted as if he had the right to deny his wife the chance to say goodbye to her brother."

Her tears abated, but not the sorrow and anger in her eyes. Sensing this was a pivotal moment for her, I asked what happened after her father's denial of her mother's plea.

"Mom changed after this incident," Sandeep said. "She seemed to be ill more often, and more demanding. And she definitely became more critical. My aunt told me that Mom loved this brother because he was the only person who showed her any kindness when she was young. I cannot imagine how heartbreaking it must have been for her to leave her brother behind in India when she moved to England with Dad. And not being allowed to see him again before he died must have killed her."

I withheld my thoughts at that moment, but couldn't stop thinking of the truth she relayed. Sandeep was correct in her assessment that this event, and others like it, had emotionally killed her mother. The severe emotional abuse she received from her parents and husband had stopped her from growing up emotionally and knowing herself as a person in her own right. All she knew about who she was, was what her parents and husband had told her. And because they told her that she was a bad housekeeper and gave her little attention and affection, Sandeep's mother was starving, hungry for any crumb of love and attention she could get. As a girl and young wife, she had tried to feel loved by being a dutiful daughter and supportive wife. But all the years of abuse and emotional neglect wore her down until she retired to bed, expecting Sandeep to take over her caregiving role and feed her emotionally starved soul, a daunting task for anyone, but especially for a daughter who was desperate to carve out her own life path.

A previous counselor Sandeep had consulted about her mother's angry, critical behavior had diagnosed her mother as suffering from a personality disorder. I was sure this diagnosis was correct. But diagnosing Sandeep's mother's maladaptive behaviors to her life of extreme emotional neglect as a mental health disorder left Sandeep with little understanding of the underlying reasons for her mother's behavior. It also created an unfair and inaccurate bias that blamed Sandeep's mother for creating her own pathology, while absolving her family from being accountable for the emotional damage their sexist beliefs had inflicted on their daughter, and on the other women in the family. And diagnosing her mother wouldn't empower Sandeep to not repeat the abuse and emotional neglect her mother and grandmother suffered.

Sandeep needed to be coached to look beyond her mother's mental health diagnosis and understand how the men in her generational family used their cultural and religious belief in the Culture of Female Service to justify how they controlled, abused, and neglected women. She needed to understand how the Culture of Female Service causes women to be emotionally starved. And she needed to recognize the symptoms of emotional starvation so she could better understand herself and her mother.

Emotional Starvation

The symptoms of emotional starvation are easy to detect, if you know what to look for. Being emotionally starved makes women too eager to please, needing too much to be liked, too fearful of being their own advocate, and prone to excessive caregiving and self-neglect. It makes women engage in attention-seeking behaviors, like being passive-aggressive, emotionally manipulative, a drama queen, and a martyr. Saying no and setting healthy boundaries is scary for emotionally starved women. This is because they need people's attention too much and they have had too many experiences of people reacting angrily when they spoke their truth. Emotional starvation also, in my experience, causes women to suffer from mental health problems like depression, anxiety, and eating disorders, because they are symptoms of women having lost their power to speak and be heard. It predisposes women to tolerate violent and abusive relationships, because they need the relationship too much. And it sets women up to feel jealous of other women who receive the attention and affection they are craving.

Ruth (the mother in Chapter 1) expressed her emotional starvation through being passive-aggressive and emotionally withdrawn. Katherine (in Chapter 2) expressed hers by overaccommodating her boyfriend's needs and tolerating how both her mother and her boyfriend abused and neglected her. Sandeep's mother used criticism, guilt-tripping, and frequent bouts of fake illness to manipulate her daughter into feeding her emotional hunger. Research shows that in families where caregiving is treated as a woman's role, women are more likely to suffer from emotional neglect. In families where women's emotional needs aren't inquired after or honored, mothers and daughters, and mothers and daughters-in-law, are set up to fight over their unvoiced and unrecognized needs. Daughters and daughters-in-law are set up to feel an exaggerated responsibility for their mother's or mother's-in-law unvoiced and neglected needs. And daughters and daughters-in-law will inevitably inherit their mother's and mother-in-law's emotional silence and emotional neglect, because they aren't exposed to a reality where their needs matter.

Changing her family's pattern of emotional neglect and emotional starvation was up to Sandeep. Escape for Sandeep's mother was unthinkable. She was too poorly educated and too emotionally damaged to think her way out of her powerlessness. And because her father and brothers were unwilling to listen to Sandeep and understand how harmful their belief in the Culture of Female Service was, she had two difficult options: She could either submit to her father's control, or fight for her freedom. She could step into her mother's shoes and walk a repeat of her mother's life, or find a different way of living where she was heard and respected. In my mind, Sandeep had only one choice to make. But that choice would mean losing her family and community, because they wouldn't tolerate her becoming a self-focused, emotionally entitled, assertive woman.

As Sandeep's therapist, it was my job to encourage her to find a way of living that supported her emotional wellbeing and emotional empowerment. As a counselor, psychotherapist, and coach, it was my duty to empower Sandeep to challenge the sexism that had harmed the women in her family and was harming her. I had to open Sandeep's eyes to a different reality, one outside the one she had learned to believe in, a reality where women were heard, emotionally supported, and treated with dignity.

Sandeep's Mother-Daughter History Map

At first Sandeep struggled to envision this new reality. She had no female role models in her family or community who had rejected the be-of-service role for women. So I took a yellow highlighter and highlighted all the emotionally neglected women on her *Mother-Daughter History Map*, so she could see how it affected every single female in her generational family. While Sandeep stared at her *Mother-Daughter History Map*—that now glowed like a Christmas tree—something clicked in place for her. She saw how women's intelligence and creativity had been deliberately discarded by her family's religious adherence to the Culture of Female Service. She saw how her dreams and emotional wellbeing were in danger of being ruined, if she continued down the path her family had set out for her. As she mused over what her mother and grandmother might have wished for, she suddenly bolted upright and asked in a puzzled voice, "Do you think Mom is making herself sick because she doesn't want me to graduate?"

I had already suspected this. Sandeep's mother's illness was too vague to be entirely physical in nature. Her bouts of sickness suspiciously coincided with Sandeep having to focus on completing an assignment or sit an exam. I've heard other daughters tell similar stories of how their mother feigned a heart attack or took to bed just when their daughter needed to focus her attention on herself. I believe that Sandeep's mother used illness to try to prevent her daughter from graduating, because she was terrified of Sandeep's growing independence. And from Sandeep's mother's perspective, I could understand her dread. Without Sandeep, she was entirely alone. But Sandeep's mother wasn't only fighting to keep her daughter emotionally and financially dependent. Having internalized the sexism that had so cruelly harmed her, she wanted Sandeep to join her in her misery. She didn't believe that Sandeep had a right to her degree, a job, and a life of her own. In her sexist and emotionally starved mind, Sandeep's mother believed that Sandeep's only purpose in life was to be of service to her mother and family.

Predictably, the stronger Sandeep became, setting boundaries with her mother and claiming her right to focus on herself, the angrier her mother became. One day Sandeep snapped when her mother called her a whore for going out with her college friends. She packed her bags and left home. She could no longer cope with her mother's unreasonable demands or be her mother's emotional punching bag.

Changing Generational Themes

Sandeep is part of a new generation of women who are eager to change their female story. She worked hard at unlearning her inherited patterns of excessive caregiving and people-pleasing. She learned how to listen for what she wanted and trust that she had a right to be heard and have her needs met. And she learned how to walk away from relationships where her needs and voice weren't welcome. At the start of her therapy, she had said she didn't want to have a daughter because she was afraid of what she would pass on to her. When we were finished, Sandeep was no longer afraid to one day be her daughter's mother. She had learned to believe in her power, and hoped to one day pass it on to her daughter.

Reflection Questionnaire: How Emotionally Hungry Are You?

This questionnaire assesses the degree of emotional silencing and emotional neglect you have been exposed to, by checking whether you are heard and visible in your relationships, and whether you're able to advocate for yourself.

Check the box that best describes how you feel about yourself at the moment, not how you think others see you.

	NEVER	SOMETIMES	MOSTLY	ALWAYS
1. I know what I need emotionally.				
2. I can advocate for what I need.				
3. I can set healthy boundaries and say no when I want to.				
4. I can tell people when I am feeling angry and hurt.				
5. I feel heard and emotionally supported by the people I love. They inquire about what I need and how I am feeling.				
6. I find it easy to talk about myself.				
7. I like who I am.				
8. I am high on my priority list.				
9. I am able to heal my emotional pain and hurtful experiences.				
10. I feel in control of my life.				

PART TWO

PUTTING THE PUZZLE TOGETHER

CHAPTER 4

A HOLISTIC MODEL THAT STRENGTHENS THE MOTHER-DAUGHTER RELATIONSHIP

How can mothers and daughters make themselves heard when historically they haven't been listened to?

NOW THAT I'VE explained how sexism is the root cause of mother-daughter relationship conflict, in this chapter and those following, I outline the *Mother-Daughter Coaching Model.* This best-practice model is a new way of understanding the dynamics between mothers and daughters. It provides mothers and daughters, and therapists, with a road-map on how to dig below the arguments mothers and daughters have. It uncovers how women's generational history, with emotional silence, denied needs, and restrictive gender roles and stereotypes, continues to harm the mother-daughter relationship. And it teaches women and therapists how to change harmful, sexist beliefs and generational patterns, and create emotionally empowered mothers and daughters who are heard, understood, and loved.

For the *Mother-Daughter Coaching Model,* I drew inspiration from family systems theory, feminist counseling theory, and psychodynamic theory. These philosophies enable women and therapists to understand the multigenerational and sociocultural nature of the mother-daughter relationship, and how the political is very personal for mothers and daughters, as depicted in the diagram below.

MOTHER-DAUGHTER PUZZLE SOLUTION

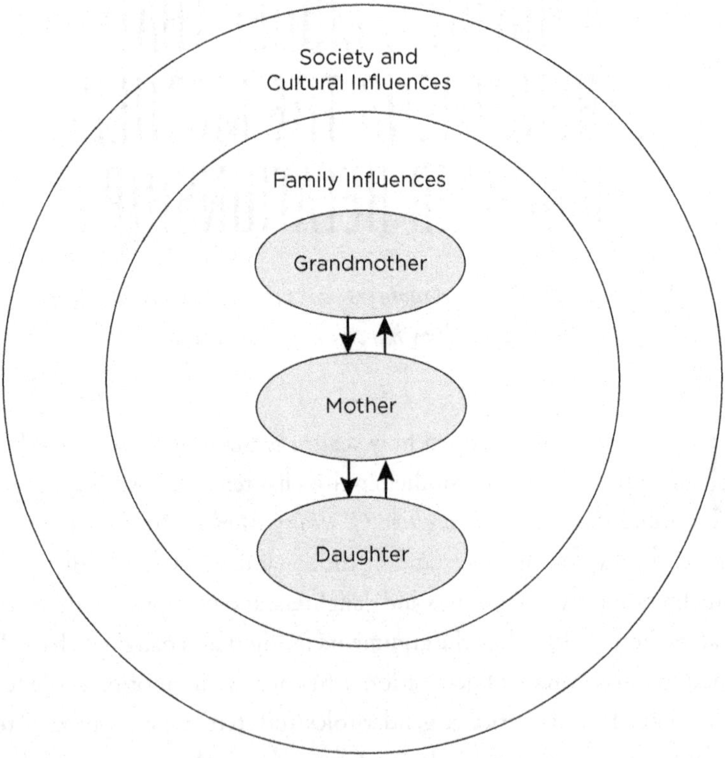

Cognitive behavioral therapy also has a voice in this model, because it teaches women how to challenge and change harmful inherited beliefs. The model is infused with the ideas and writing of feminists like Paula Caplan, Betty Friedan, Susie Orbach, Andrea O'Reilly, Adrienne Rich, and Gloria Steinem, to name a few, who know that empowering mothers and daughters is central to women's fight for equal rights. The model has been informed by women's development theorists like Carol Gilligan, Lyn Mikel Brown, Jean Baker Miller, and many others who have studied women's development, and how patriarchy silences women.

I have deliberately made the *Mother-Daughter Coaching Model* accessible to everyone, not just therapists with a psychology or psychotherapy degree. I want all women to benefit from what I have learned, and to use the three solutions that are explained below. In summary, the three solutions teach mothers and daughters of all ages how to uncover the core reasons for their arguments; how to feel entitled to voice their feelings, thoughts, and needs; how to map their mother-daughter history; and how to create generational change.

Solution 1: Mothers Are People First

This solution exposes one of the main causes of mother-daughter conflict—our deep-seated belief in the Culture of Female Service. And it reveals how some therapeutic modalities and human development theories that mental health professionals use are based on the sexist notion that women and mothers are caregivers, with little to no identity as people in their own right.

I saw this bias on display at Nottingham University, during a talk by Sir Richard Bowlby, son of the late Sir John Bowlby, who was the father of attachment theory. *Attachment theory* is a psychological model that describes how babies bond with their parents, and how feeling secure in this relationship is essential for their emotional development. During Sir Richard's talk, he presented slide after slide of what he interpreted as traumatized babies being handed over by their mothers to childcare workers at daycare centers. He had selected photos of grim-looking, wide-eyed babies to prove his point that mothers are traumatizing their babies when they send them to a childminder. He didn't show any slide of a happy baby being handed over to its childminder or a father handing over his baby to childminders. He also didn't speak about why mothers, and fathers, need to use childcare for their children.

Sir Richard is correct in his teaching that babies and young children need to bond with their caregiver for their emotional development. What he isn't correct about, and caused the mothers in the lecture to feel unnecessary guilt over, is how he used subliminal messaging to reinforce the sexist belief that mothers are the only and best caregivers of babies. In my work with mothers and daughters, I see on a daily basis how this myopic view of motherhood creates the following five problems.

First: Mother-Blaming

Sir Richard Bowlby's views feed right into patriarchy's proclivity to blame mothers. Sadly, he is far from alone with his mother-blaming message. In the book *The New Don't Blame Mother*, Paula Caplan writes that mother-blaming is a widespread form of prejudice. When she reviewed professional journals for references to mothers being blamed for causing their children harm, she found that mothers were being blamed for an eye-watering range of problems like bed wetting, troubled teenagers, schizophrenia, learning problems, homosexuality, and eating disorders.[1] This culture of mother-blaming extends to pathologizing mothers whose emotional health is suffering from not having a life or identity outside of their mothering role. During my mother's generation, doctors prescribed depressed mothers Valium, commonly called "mother's little helper." Today, the medical profession uses a much larger range of drugs to medicate mothers who are screaming for an identity of their own.

Second: Stress and Exhaustion

The view of mothers as the "ideal" caregiver shames mothers into neglecting themselves, setting them up for exhaustion and stress. Allison Pearson, author of *I Don't Know How She Does It*, bravely admitted to *The Guardian* how she suffered from depression due to her crazy juggling act of trying to meet her family and job responsibilities. I agree with the article's assessment, that depression amongst mothers is the curse of the modern mother who tries to "have it all" by "doing it all."[2] But I also think this problem has deeper roots than women wanting to "have it all." It is rooted in our belief that caregiving is a female behavior and not a human behavior. It's also a symptom of how emotional neglect is the bedrock on which mothers have mothered for generations, and still do today.

Third: Emotional Neglect

Following from the concept that emotional neglect is the bedrock on which mothers mother, my clients show me how this mothering experience causes some mothers to be overavailable and superattentive toward their daughter. This dynamic happens for two main reasons. First, mothers don't want their daughters to know how horrible it feels to be neglected. And second, they hope this "overavailable, superattentive" approach will stop their daughter from inheriting their own experiences of emotional neglect.

The sad truth is, this dynamic creates an imbalanced mother-daughter relationship, where what the daughter needs outweighs what the mother needs. Whenever a mother tolerates being neglected and neglects herself, she is teaching her daughter how to live a life of neglect. Every time she silences herself and allows herself to be last on the list, she is showing her daughter that emotional silence and neglect are normal for women. And when her daughter becomes a mother, she will in all likelihood mother her children in the same self-neglecting and self-sacrificing way she herself was mothered. And so the pattern of emotional neglect and lack of personal identity carries on into the next generation.

Fourth: Daughters Meeting Their Mothers' Unmet Needs

As Sandeep's story revealed in Chapter 3, emotional neglect sets daughters up to provide the emotional care their mother isn't receiving or giving to herself. When mothers don't matter as people, a dynamic I call "the river of nurturing flowing backwards up the generations" is created. In healthy families, where women's needs and voices are inquired after and heard, nurturing flows easily down the generations from mother to daughter. But in families where women aren't heard and emotionally supported, daughters, and often eldest daughters, are given the role of meeting their mother's denied emotional needs. This means that the flow of nurturing flows backwards, up the generations, rather than down the generations, leaving the daughter to focus on what her mother needs rather than what she needs.

This pattern of reverse nurturing ensures that the experience of emotional neglect and emotional starvation is passed on to the daughter. In her role as her mother's emotional caregiver, the daughter learns to become an expert on what her mother needs, rather than on what she herself needs, which stops her from learning how to speak the language that inquires after and values what she needs. This dynamic will directly affect the daughter's other relationships, as she views herself, and is viewed by others, as someone whose main function is to be of service, rather than a human who needs and deserves care and attention so she can flourish.

Fifth: Payback Mothers, Stepmothers, and Grandmothers

Finally, emotionally neglected mothers are in danger of becoming what I call "payback mothers" or "payback mothers-in-law." Payback mothers are women, usually in their sixties or seventies, who have become exhausted and given-out after a lifetime of service. They stop giving of themselves and pass the baton of caregiving on to a daughter, or daughter-in-law, not a son or son-in-law, and expect her to "pay her back" for all the care and attention she has given over her lifetime by being super-attentive to her mother's or mother-in-law's needs.

Even though being a payback mother or mother-in-law is highly manipulative, within the context of a lifetime of selfless service, it makes sense. It is human to become depleted if you haven't been taught how to replenish the emotional bucket from which you give. The boundaries daughters and daughters-in-law have to put in place so they don't inherit their mother's, or mother-in-law's, self-neglect and become the next generation of payback mothers do little to address the confusion payback mothers and mothers-in-law feel when their investment in their family doesn't pay out in the way they had hoped. It's important that daughters and daughters-in-law remember that they will never be able to make up for the neglect their mother or mother-in-law experienced. They must focus their attention on learning how to take care of themselves and changing the conversation within their family so that mothers and daughters matter as people from now on.

Solution 2: The Mother-Daughter Relationship Is Lifelong

This solution refutes how the media and counseling and human development theories often marginalize the mother-daughter relationship into single-issue problems, such as a mother with her "troubled" teenage daughter, or an adult daughter with a "difficult" elderly mother. My research shows that the mother-daughter relationship is a lifelong relationship, made up of eight distinct stages that reflect the mother's and daughter's individual growth and development. I find that clients typically call for help when they're struggling to navigate a particular stage in their relationship. Issues and conflicts that weren't resolved when the daughter was an adolescent, for example, often bubble up to the surface at a later stage, demanding to be healed. Each stage requires that mothers and daughters respond to their individual developmental issues, which I outline below. On a general note, each stage requires that mothers and daughters renew their learning of how to better listen to and understand each other, create a mutually supportive relationship when the daughter is an adult, and reject sexist and restrictive gender roles and stereotypes.

The Daughter Is Born

Becoming your daughter's mother is, as Elizabeth Debold, Marie Wilson, and Idelisse Malave write in *Mother Daughter Revolution*, "one of the most powerful and the most political" moments in a woman's life.[3] It provides a mother with an opportunity to be a catalyst for change and facilitate an emotionally empowered future for her daughter.

Facilitating this emotionally empowered future for your daughter starts with challenging your internalized Culture of Female Service. It starts with challenging the sexism in your generational family that silences women's voices and sets mothers and daughters up to battle over their respective emotional silence and emotional starvation. This means that a mother needs to see herself as a person first. She needs to seize her entitlement to have a life and identity outside her role as mother, and be emotionally honest about what she feels, thinks, and needs. As she creates this emotional reality for herself, she will be passing this new normal on to her daughter, who will learn to expect that as a woman she deserves to be heard and emotionally supported.

The Daughter Is an Adolescent

During this stage, mothers and daughters hit head-on against the multigenerational impact of sexism. The sudden spike in mother-daughter relationship conflict when daughters enter puberty isn't caused by teenage hormones, as is commonly believed. It is caused by adolescent girls slamming up against "the wall," as Carol Gilligan calls it, of their families, and society's, patriarchal beliefs.[4]

During adolescence, patriarchy intensifies its pressure on girls to comply with its "good girl" role model. As I wrote in *The Silent Female Scream*, "The definition of a 'good girl' hasn't changed much since our grandmother's day. It still means fitting in, fitting around, giving in to what others want us to do, and definitely not upsetting anyone."[5] And, to add insult upon injury, patriarchy charges mothers with the task of socializing their daughters to be "good girls." It's not surprising that this causes conflict between mothers and their adolescent daughters. Daughters are set up to vent their anger at having to silence themselves at their mother, because it's hard to rage at an unquantifiable, impersonal social system that is afraid of women being too vocal and too demanding. And in families where the father is either emotionally unavailable or absent, mothers are again set up to bear the brunt of a daughter's anger about her father's abandonment.

One of the difficulties in recognizing these underlying dynamics is that adolescent daughters often voice their anger about having to fit in and keep quiet in a dysfunctional or emotionally withdrawn way. In my work with mothers and adolescent daughters, I help them decode the daughter's behavior, helping connect the dots between the daughter's difficult or argumentative behavior and the way their family prioritizes male voices over female voices and emotionally neglects women. I find that when mothers and daughters make these connections, their arguments start to make more sense, and they are empowered to join together to challenge the sexism in their family.

This leads to another dynamic, one at the heart of mother and adolescent-daughter conflict. Carol Gilligan, Lyn Mikel Brown, Jean Baker Miller, and the researchers at the Stone Center, Wellesley College, discovered that adolescent daughters are wired to emotionally mature through their emotional connection with their mother.[6] I have found this to be true with daughters of all ages, who look to their mothers for answers about who they are and what it means to be female. These findings contradict many developmental theories that assume young daughters need to emotionally separate from their mothers for their growth and development. In all my years of listening to mothers and daughters talk about their relationships, I have yet to meet a mother-daughter couple who isn't fighting to remain emotionally connected. Underneath their arguments lies an emotional hunger to feel known by each other. The only reason a daughter might need to emotionally separate from her mother is when her mother is abusive, and remaining in the relationship endangers the daughter's self-worth and emotional wellbeing, as Sandeep's story in Chapter 3 showed.

The Daughter Leaves Home and Becomes an Adult

At this stage, the mother-daughter relationship changes from an adult-child relationship to an adult-adult or woman-to-woman relationship, where their relationship has to move to being more mutually supportive. This means that the flow of caring and support needs to flow both ways, and a daughter can no longer expect her mother to drop whatever she's doing whenever the daughter needs her, if that's what she was used to as a child. An adult daughter needs to know who her mother is as a person and woman, because this helps her understand herself.

At this time, it's important that mothers and daughters talk about how they feel about their physical separation and their excitement about their newfound freedoms. Mothers need to reflect on the changes in their mothering role and be encouraged to awaken old dreams. Any jealousy a mother might feel about her daughter's freedom and potential should be talked about and understood. (It's important to note that it isn't only mothers who can feel jealous. I have worked with many daughters who felt jealous of their mother's creativity or their mother's courage to go for what she wants.)

The Daughter Gets Married or Chooses a Life Partner

Many mothers and daughters seek help at this stage because a daughter's wedding can bring up old power struggles as well as unresolved maternal jealousy. In families where women receive little attention and few celebrations, a wedding puts tremendous pressure on a daughter to claim her one day in the limelight. And if a mother has spent her life living in the shadows, it can be hard for her to watch her daughter get the attention and celebration she herself had to forego. Conventional wisdom often dismisses this kind of maternal jealousy as petty. It isn't. It is real, and if honored, it empowers mothers and daughters to create a new normal for the women in their family.

This stage also heralds the daughter's relationship with her mother-in-law. Mothers and daughters-in-law are set up for conflict in the same way mothers and daughters are. How the mother-in-law has been treated by her family, whether she is heard or emotionally silenced, emotionally supported or emotionally neglected, has been encouraged to realize her dreams or forced to fit into restrictive gender roles, and is dealing with internalized sexism, all will impact how she relates to her daughter-in-law.

I recommend that mothers and daughters-in-law spend time together mapping the mother-in-law's mother-daughter history. This exercise will help the daughter-in-law understand who her mother-in-law is, and how her life experiences and themes in her generational family will influence how she views her daughter-in-law. Even better if the daughter's new husband participates in this exercise. He needs to bear witness to his mother's life, and the beliefs and gender stereotypes he has grown up with and internalized. But if the mother-in-law isn't willing to participate, I suggest that the daughter-in-law and her new husband map out what they know about his mother's mother-daughter history, so they can identify the beliefs and gender stereotypes they need to change.

I'd like to mention the issue of a daughter, or mother, being lesbian. This issue is a difficult one for mothers and daughters to navigate when they come from a homophobic family or from a family that adheres to traditional gender roles. It also hits against the dynamic I mention in Chapter 2 where some mothers and daughters need to see themselves reflected in each other's lives. As with all the life stages, this issue requires that a mother and daughter learn how to listen to and accept each other's differences and uniqueness, and that they join in resisting their family's prejudice so it doesn't have the power to divide them.

The Daughter Becomes a Mother and the Mother a Grandmother

At this life stage, the mother-daughter relationship expands to include a new daughter. As I explain in Hannah and Ruth's story in Chapter 1, the daughter, as a new mom, will need to reflect on how she was mothered by her mother, as part of her learning about how she wants to mother her new daughter. This examination can spark hurtful conflict if the daughter feels that her mother's mothering was lacking. And the mother, as she watches her daughter become a mother, will reflect on what it was like for her when she was a new mom, and how different it was for her back then.

Babies are demanding, and daughters need all the help and emotional support they can get from their mothers. But in families that don't emotionally support women, this stage can be a struggle. An unsupported, emotionally starved mother might not understand what her daughter needs, and the daughter might not know how to ask for what she needs. For some clients, I suggest they make a pact that for the next six months the focus of their relationship will be on what the daughter needs, within reason—no mother can be expected to leave work or put her life on hold just because her daughter has a baby. For this pact to work, the daughter will need to learn how to ask for what she needs and not expect her mom to be a mind reader. When the six months is up, they will have to work on reverting to a more mutually supportive relationship.

One issue that can rear its head at this stage is how some grandmothers find it easier to be emotionally supportive toward their granddaughter than they did their daughter. This dynamic is extremely painful for the adult daughter. It is hard to watch your daughter receive the love and attention you never got from your mother. The jealousy a mother feels toward her daughter is entirely natural and understandable. But if this dynamic lies hidden and unresolved, it has the power to increase the conflict between the adult daughter and her mother. It can also harm the daughter's relationship with her young daughter, and sabotage the young daughter's relationship with her grandmother. In these cases, I help the adult daughter grieve her very normal feelings of loss about what she will never receive from her mother. I help her understand, through mapping her mother-daughter history, why her mother was, or is, emotionally unavailable for her. And I help her understand that her mother did the best she could with the little she received, even though it wasn't good enough for her. I also explain how the grandmother-granddaughter relationship is different from the mother-daughter relationship. Grandmothers do not expect their granddaughters to meet their unmet and unvoiced needs in the same way they expect this of their daughters.

The Mother Enters Menopause

Menopause can be a difficult time for women, both physically and emotionally. Yet underneath the hot flashes and hormonal fluctuations is a wonderful opportunity for mothers to prioritize their needs and life goals, often for the first time. I have worked with many amazing women who during this time got divorced, started a business, and said no for the first time. And when their family reacted negatively against their boldness, they didn't buckle under their family's pressure to return to their be-of-service gender role. These mothers showed their daughters, through their actions, that women can be masters of their own destiny. Among the mothers I've counseled, one took up road biking, another learned to trust her body through her fight with cancer, and another left an abusive husband.

The Elderly Mother

During this stage, the caregiving role is reversed; the daughter takes care of her physically dependent mother. The loss of independence can be difficult for mothers, especially if they haven't accepted that it is human to have needs. This stage is also the last opportunity for mothers and daughters to repair and strengthen their relationship. Caring for an elderly mother is extra difficult when a daughter hasn't been mothered enough, and the mother is critical and demanding. The daughter will need to reconcile with the reality that she will never have the mother she needs, and find a way to understand and accept the mother she has. She will also need to separate herself from her mother's criticism or emotional blackmail. She will need to understand that her mother's hurtful behaviors are a symptom of her mother's emotional starvation, not a reflection of her as a daughter. And it is imperative that the daughter sets clear boundaries about what she can and cannot provide for her mother, so she doesn't inherit or repeat her mother's selflessness and self-sacrifice. Daughters in this situation must demand that other siblings and family members, including males, take responsibility for their equal share in taking care of Mom. If family members refuse to help out, I suggest that my clients invoice them for the time they're unwilling to provide.

The Mother Dies

Saying goodbye to a much-loved mother is heartbreaking enough on its own. A daughter needs to give herself all the time she needs to grieve the loss of her beloved mother and find a way of honoring her life. And for daughters who had a difficult relationship with their mothers, a mother's death can bring up unresolved pain and anger. I find that society's religiously based message that daughters should forgive their abusive and neglecting mothers as hurtful, toxic, guilt producing (see Chapter 8 for an explanation of what toxic guilt is), and unhelpful to the healing process. Women need a world where both the mother's emotional reality and the daughter's truth about her relationship with her mother have an equal voice. This voice needs to understand, and have empathy for, how a mother's own experiences of abuse, emotional starvation, or emotional neglect led her to be abusive and neglectful toward her daughter. And it needs to have an equally valid understanding of how the mother's hurtful and abusive behavior damaged her daughter's emotional wellbeing. This conversation needs to honor the way a mother was damaged by the sexism in her generation and the abuse she experienced, and how this damage was repeated in the way she mothered her daughter. Through these kinds of conversations, mothers and daughters will be heard and understood, and harmful generational patterns changed forever.

Solution 3: The Mother-Daughter Relationship Is A History Lesson

This solution challenges the incorrect assumption that the mother-daughter relationship is a self-contained dyad. Research shows that history repeats itself between mothers and daughters, especially when mothers and daughters don't share the stories of what has happened to the women in their generational family, and how their lives and self-worth have been emotionally affected by the way their family and culture treats women. I see repeatedly how eating disorders, depression, anxiety disorders, violence, and sexual abuse, as well as emotional silencing and emotional neglect, are multigenerational issues. These daughters unconsciously repeat the abuse from which their mothers suffered, inherit their mothers' dieting behaviors and body hatred, and generation after generation, keep marrying men who are emotionally unavailable.

I've seen the time-tested maxim "We repeat what we don't understand" through my own life, and my clients' lives. Without knowing it or wanting to, as a young wife and mother during the 1980s and 1990s, I repeated the same emotional neglect and invisibility my mother suffered from. As a teenager, I hated seeing how bored and unhappy my mother looked as she walked to the corner shop each day to get the day's groceries. At the time I thought her boredom and unhappiness came from her not having a job and identity outside her role as mother and wife. So when I heard the feminist cry of "have it all," which gave mothers and wives permission to juggle their career along with their family responsibilities, I thought I had found the answer I had been looking for.

At the time, I believed that walking a different life from my mother's meant following my career goals. I thought that if I claimed an identity outside my role as mother and wife, I wouldn't end up depressed and angry like her. So when my children were babies, I enrolled, as a part-time student, in the Bachelor of Education degree program at the University of Canterbury, New Zealand. When my family and I later moved to England and I set up my private psychotherapy practice specializing in the mother-daughter relationship, I fitted my work around my children's school day.

But as my mother-daughter relationship work developed, and I mapped my own mother-daughter history, I was shocked to discover how much I had repeated my mother's life. Underneath our different façades and my increased options and opportunities lay the same themes I saw in every client's *Mother-Daughter History Map* I drew. Like most women, I had inadvertently repeated the emotional silence and emotional neglect my mother, and grandmother, had suffered from. I saw that a lack of job or career, though a contributing factor, wasn't the root cause of my mother's unhappiness. Her depression and anger came from a much deeper emotional reality, one that revealed how my multigenerational family emotionally silenced and emotionally neglected women. And despite my outward appearance of living a more feminist and empowered life, I too was emotionally silent and tolerating unacceptable levels of emotional neglect in my marriage, and other relationships.

It was hard to grasp how my idea of juggling my career with caring for my family hadn't changed my inherited emotional legacy. I hated seeing how I too had been bored and unhappy, even as I walked my children to preschool and school each day. How I had selected college classes, not because I was interested in them, but because they were at a time when my husband and his parents were available to babysit the children. How I had squeezed my study time into the spaces when my children were asleep, so they and my husband were in no way inconvenienced by my need to study. How I had set my hours of my private psychotherapy practice to fit in with my children's school day, because I didn't feel entitled to claim whatever time I needed for my work. And that I had married into a family that was similar to mine, in the way it emotionally neglected wives and mothers through its strict adherence to the Culture of Female Service.

It took some time for me to understand that, even though my mother's controlling behavior gave that appearance, my mother didn't know how to advocate for herself, or how to make space for herself in her marriage and relationships. Like me, she didn't know how to voice what she needed in an open and honest way. And neither of us had a core *knowing* that we had a right to be heard, nurtured, and emotionally supported.

I also uncovered an interesting fact through mapping my mother-daughter history. The women in my family tended to emigrate during their twenties or early thirties. My great-grandmother emigrated to Indonesia during her twenties, so her husband could take up his post as a missionary. My grandmother returned to Indonesia during her twenties, to be back with her mother after having spent her childhood growing up in Holland. My mother emigrated to New Zealand when she was twenty-seven. I moved to America when I was thirty. And because of this, all these women have lived, and my daughter and I are still living, in a different country from the one where we were born. My great-grandmother was born in Holland, and she lived out her entire adult life in Indonesia. My grandmother was born in Indonesia, and she lived the last part of her life in New Zealand. My mother was born in Indonesia, and she lived out her life in New Zealand. I was born in New Zealand and I am now living in America. And my daughter was born in New Zealand, and she now lives in England.

This is an important theme to acknowledge, not only because it is a curious coincidence, but also because it tells a story of how the women in my family have had to emotionally adjust to different cultures and countries, and how this affected their mother-daughter relationships. It also tells the story of women's autonomy or lack of autonomy through the exploration of why we each moved countries. Did we move because that was what we wanted, or was it to follow our husband or father?

After the initial shock about the emotional truth of my life wore off, I started to feel stronger. I now had answers to questions that had troubled me for a long time. And I knew what I needed to change so my daughter didn't inherit my emotional silence and emotional neglect. As I repeatedly teach in my workshops, when it comes to understanding ourselves as women, all roads lead to understanding our mother's and grandmother's lives, as the diagram at the start of this chapter shows. Strengthening yourself emotionally as a woman, and understanding who you are and why you make the choices you do, starts with understanding what you have inherited from your mother. The same is true for therapists. For therapists to truly understand their female clients, they need to understand what happened to the women in previous generations, particularly whether they were heard or silenced, emotionally supported or emotionally neglected, and how their generation's gender roles and stereotypes limited their choices.

When women learn about their mother's and grandmother's lives and the emotional reality they lived in, women are learning about themselves. When women honor the sacrifices their mothers and grandmothers have had to make, they are learning about the emotional consequences of sacrifice and the intelligence and creativity that have been lost through centuries of sexism. When women respect the courage, resilience, and wisdom their mothers and grandmothers showed, they are connecting with their own. Whenever I feel unsure about whether I can do something, I remember how my silent, submissive grandmother had the courage to stand up to the invading Japanese soldiers in Indonesia during the Second World War. The story told in my family tells of how my grandmother hid stolen medicine in her laundry basket, moments before the Japanese soldiers marched through her house looking for it. When I think about how she risked death if found out, because she believed that the medicine needed to be used fairly, by whoever needed it, regardless of whether they were an invading Japanese soldier, colonial Dutch resident, or Indonesian, I know that I can do whatever I need to do.

When my colleagues and I use the concepts in the *Mother-Daughter Coaching Model*, women's history and the mother-daughter relationship are pulled away from the margins and restored to their rightful place, front and center in women's lives. Mother-daughter conflicts, which seemed confusing before, start to make sense as mothers and daughters learn to speak and understand each other's emotional truths. And with the exposure of how emotional silence and emotional neglect are the cornerstone of sexism and gender inequality, and how they harm women's emotional wellbeing, mother-daughter relationships and all relationships, and women's equality and human rights, women are fortified to create an emotionally empowered future for themselves and their daughters.

By now you might be thinking you would like to know more about your own mother-daughter history, based on the benefits of knowing what I have described here. Or perhaps that's why you picked up this book—to seek to understand some difficulty in your own mother-daughter relationship. In the next two chapters I describe the theory behind, and give detailed instructions on, how you can map *your* mother-daughter history.

Reflection Questionnaire: How Strong Is Your Mother and Adult-Daughter Relationship?

This questionnaire assesses the health of your relationship with your mother/adult-daughter. Check the box that best describes how *you* are feeling about your relationship with your mother/adult daughter at the moment.

I suggest that you and your mother/daughter complete the questionnaire on your own first, and then compare results.

	NEVER	SOMETIMES	MOSTLY	ALWAYS
1. I can be honest and say what I'm feeling without feeling guilty.				
2. My privacy is respected.				
3. I am free to make my own decisions and mistakes.				
4. My decisions and boundaries are respected.				
5. I am encouraged and supported to grow and change.				
6. My relationship with my mother/daughter has changed to incorporate my growth.				
7. When we disagree, my opinions and feelings are treated with equal importance.				
8. I feel heard.				
9. I enjoy my mother's/daughter's company.				
10. I take responsibility for my needs and choices.				

CHAPTER 5

REALIZING THE POWER IN YOUR MOTHER-DAUGHTER HISTORY

Imagine a world where what women need rolls off the tongue with ease, and we no longer remember that there was a time when this conversation didn't exist.

TWENTY YEARS AGO, when I was a young therapist, I learned how powerful it is to draw a client's family tree or *genogram*, as it is called in family systems therapy. Family trees are a great way of recording what has happened in a woman's generational family, including the gender roles that women and men have had to live by, the jobs and careers they had, any physical and emotional health issues, and whether they were/are kind or abusive toward each other. But early on, the conventional way I was taught to draw a client's family tree started to frustrate me. It seemed to lack a clear female voice. I felt that women's emotional reality often remained hidden behind male voices and gender stereotypes. To me, a family tree that didn't tell the unfiltered truth of a woman's life and the emotional experience of what it means to be female in her generational family was colluding with, and perpetuating, the silencing and invisibility of women.

So I decided I had to go on a quest to find a new way of drawing women's female history, so that they told the bold, unfiltered truth about how women feel about their lives. I wanted to find a way to draw a woman's female history, so she could see how her mother-daughter relationship was affected by the changes in women's roles, women's multigenerational experience with sexism, the dark underbelly of the Culture of Female Service, and the marginalization of the mother-daughter relationship. I wanted women to understand how the experiences of emotional silence, emotional neglect, and emotional abuse, to name a few, are passed down from mother to daughter. I wanted women to own the courage and strength inherent in women's psyches. And I wanted to give my clients a plan of action that provided the tools they needed to create emotionally empowered lives and mutually supportive, gender-equal relationships, and challenge harmful sexist beliefs and cultural practices.

Isabella was the inspiration for the *Mother-Daughter History Mapping* exercise I use today. She made me realize that I needed to exclude men's stories and men's needs from my multigenerational map, because they were hindering my ability to hear women's emotional reality clearly. Isabella was a sixteen-year-old schoolgirl who had been ordered to see me by her father, because he wanted me to "cure" her from her disruptive behaviors. Her father believed that Isabella's belligerent behavior and extreme dieting were signs of her mental instability.

Isabella was a petite girl with long, straight brown hair. When I first met her, she wore thick makeup and her hair hung loose over her face, which reminded me of a mask behind which she needed to hide. At first, her therapy was slow going because she didn't trust me. She resented that her father had ordered her to see me, and she thought I was there to follow her father's instructions and "cure" her from her rebellious behavior. After a few sessions where Isabella sat in silence, refusing to engage with any of my questions, I asked her if she was willing to draw out her family tree. I was hoping this exercise would be less threatening to her, and I wanted to find out what was going on in her family.

Thankfully Isabella was interested, and she immediately launched into stories about the men in her family. She told me her grandfather had been a violent man, and that her uncle had been in a psychiatric hospital a number of times for physically abusing his wife. As I listened to her stories of the violence in her family, something snapped inside me. I couldn't listen to her anymore, and I couldn't draw out her family tree unless we started to focus on the women.

In a split-second decision, I did something radical. I decided to throw out the rules and create a new way of drawing a woman's family tree. Not having had time to prepare myself for this sudden change in tack, I decided to throw caution to the wind and tell Isabella what I was feeling. I told her that I was frustrated with how women tend to focus on what's happening in men's lives rather than their own. That I want to hear about Isabella's life and her mother's and grandmother's lives. I wanted to hear what she thought, not what her father thought. I wanted to know what she imagined it was like for her grandmother and aunt to be married to violent men, and why neither of them got divorced. And I wanted to wake women up to the invisibility they had learned to tolerate, by drawing family trees that told the uncensored, uncontaminated, emotional truth about women's lives.

To my surprise, Isabella agreed with me. Then she told me that she didn't talk about her mother because there was nothing to say about her. "Mom is a caring person," she said, "but she does what Dad wants. She sides with him all the time, which really pisses me off. No one really talks about her, and they don't really talk about Grandma either. All the fun stories in my family are about my crazy grandfather and uncle."

I asked Isabella if she was willing to do an experiment and redraw her family tree with women only. She agreed, and in that brave, bold moment, Isabella and I gave birth to the *Mother-Daughter History Mapping* exercise. Following is a condensed version of her mapping session, with corresponding diagrams. See the end of this chapter for the complete diagram of Isabella's *Mother-Daughter History Map*.

I decided to retain the way women are drawn as a circle and men as a square, as with traditional family trees or genograms, and started by drawing three big circles vertically down the center of the page to represent the three central women in Isabella's family. I put Isabella in the bottom circle as the daughter, her mother, Cynthia, in the middle circle, and her grandmother, Ilene, in the top circle.

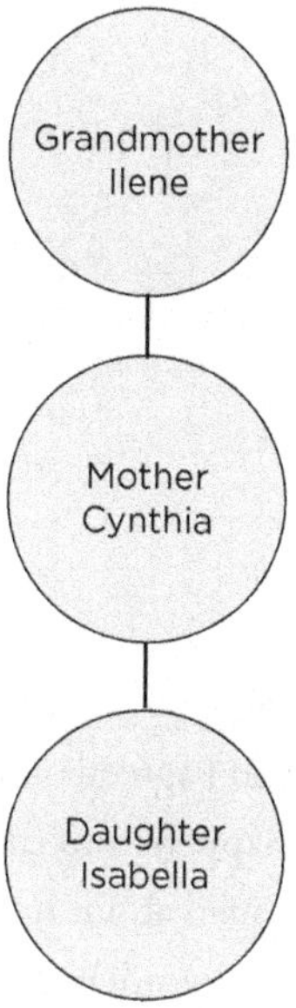

On the right side of the page I added Isabella's and Cynthia's siblings, adding Isabella's brother, Colin, and Cynthia's sister Candice. And below Auntie Candice, I added her violent husband in a square. On the left side of the page I added the men in Isabella's multigenerational family, adding her father to the left of her mother, and her grandfather to the left of her grandmother.

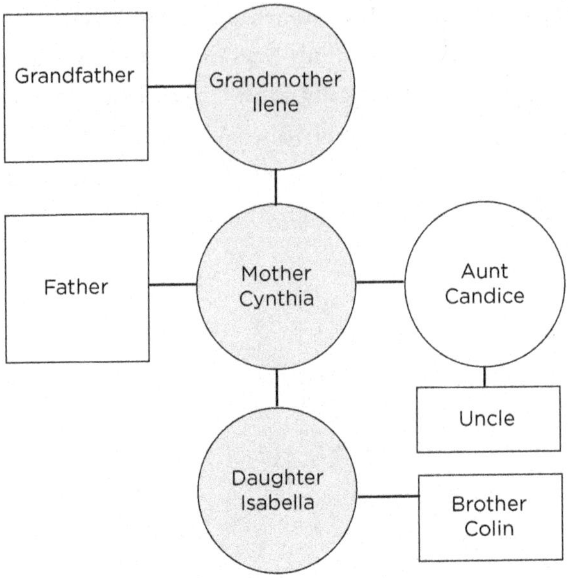

©2010 Rosjke Hasseldine

After I had finished mapping out these key people in Isabella's multi-generational family, Isabella and I agreed on two rules. First, we were only going to focus on what had happened to the women in her family. This meant that the stories we mapped about her father and grandfather had to reflect how they treated the women. And second, because this was Isabella's map, it had to reflect Isabella's unfiltered and unedited truth. It had to record what she thought about herself and the people in her family, and not what her parents thought was true about Isabella, or what her parents and grandparents believed about themselves. This is an important feature of *Mother-Daughter History Mapping*, which I explain in more detail in Chapter 6.

I started the mapping process with some facts that Isabella knew about herself, her mother, and her grandmother. In *Mother-Daughter History Maps*, I separate out the facts about women's lives from women's emotional reality. Facts include women's ages, when someone died, their occupations, and the gender roles that define the women's lives.

Emotional reality includes whether women were heard or silenced, whether women's emotional needs were honored, or denied, and what emotional health issues the women struggled with. Facts are recorded around the outside of a woman's circle; each woman's emotional reality is recorded inside her circle.

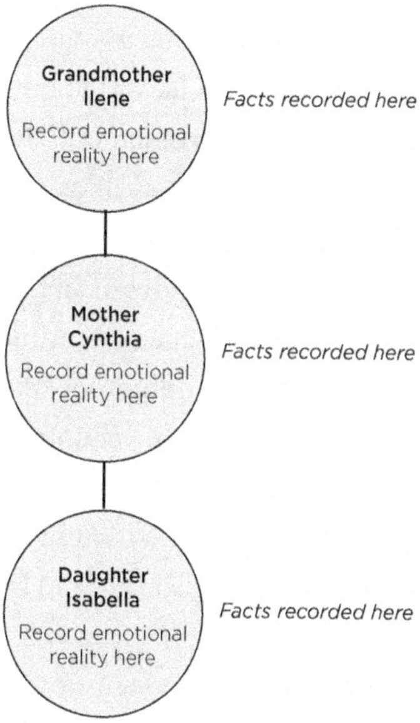

The facts we recorded for Isabella were that she was a sixteen-year-old schoolgirl who was expected to be a dutiful, obedient daughter. For her mother, Cynthia, we recorded that she was fifty-five years old, worked part-time as a secretary, and was the family caregiver. For her grandmother, Ilene, we recorded that she had died two years before, and was a homemaker all her married life and the family's caregiver.

Recording the facts was the easy part. As with many women, recalling what their emotional reality is, and what they believe their mother's and grandmother's emotional reality was, took some time. As I encouraged Isabella to look below the stories she knew about her mother and grandmother and uncover whether she, her mother, and her grandmother ever voiced what they felt, needed, and wanted, we discovered that all three women did not know how to voice what they needed, which I recorded as "no needs voice" in each of their circles. Isabella said she had never heard her mother or grandmother ask for anything for themselves, and she felt angry that no one asked her what she wanted. She said, "No one asks me what I want. Everyone behaves as if they know what I want, but they don't. They only want me to want what they want, which really means what Dad wants me to do, and I hate that."

I recorded how all three women in Isabella's family were invisible. I added how Isabella described herself as angry, how she described her mother as submissive, and how she said that her grandmother had been critical and demanding, especially of her daughter Cynthia, Isabella's mother. As Isabella looked at her emerging map, she saw, for the first time, how she, her mother, and grandmother weren't all that different from each other. She saw how her anger, her mother's submissive behavior, and her grandmother's critical behavior were all symptoms of their shared invisibility. The only difference was that her mother had decided to react in a passive way against being silenced, and Isabella and her grandmother had become critical and angry.

When we talked about any emotional struggles Isabella and her mother and grandmother suffered from, Isabella made another striking connection. She saw that her extreme dieting was an inherited behavior from her mother, who was always on one diet or another, and her aunt Candice was also a yo-yo dieter.

These kinds of connections are what *Mother-Daughter History Mapping* is designed to facilitate. It empowers women to connect the dots between how they behave, the choices they make, and the truth they have come to believe about themselves, with how their family treats women. It helped Isabella connect the dots between the theme of dieting in her multigenerational family and the extreme emotional neglect from which the women suffer.

I often see dieting behaviors and eating disorders in families where women aren't heard or emotionally supported. Eating disorders and dieting behaviors are a metaphor for the emotional starvation women experience. When women are emotionally starved, they take out this emotional reality on themselves by denying themselves the food they need to satisfy their hunger. Feeling physically hungry becomes a way of coping with emotional hunger, because physical hunger is the one thing they know how to control.

At this point in Isabella's mapping session, the conversation turned to the men in the family and how fathers and husbands treated the women they love. We started by adding a few facts around the outside of her father's square, recording that he was a busy lawyer and good provider. Isabella then described her father as a controlling, verbally abusive man, and that her grandfather was the same, which I recorded inside their respective squares. We recorded that Aunt Candice's husband was violent. I then asked her about her brother, Colin, and Isabella responded by saying, "He's exactly like Dad. He's a selfish person who only thinks about himself."

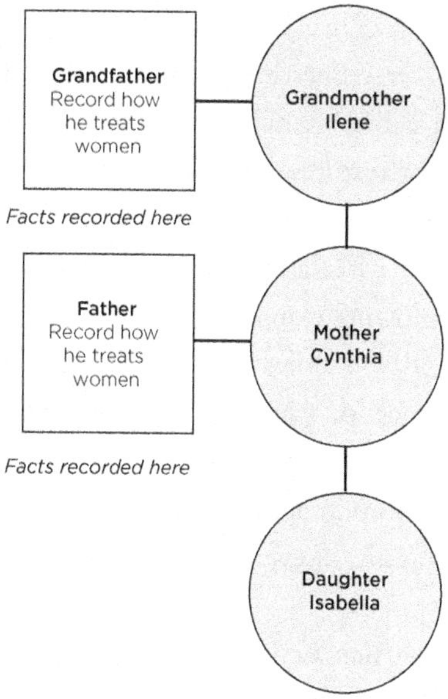

It was shocking to see how Isabella's multigenerational experience was dominated by controlling, violent men, and how Isabella's mother had repeated her mother's life. Seeing her inherited emotional reality all written out helped Isabella understand why she was so angry. Being angry was a perfectly normal reaction to the emotional silencing, emotional neglect, invisibility, and abuse that surrounded her. Isabella was angry with her father for being abusive, and with her mother for tolerating it.

While Isabella continued looking at her *Mother-Daughter History Map*, her face lit up. Blinking at tears, she said, "So I'm not crazy?"

"No you're not crazy," I replied. "It's your family that's crazy for emotionally neglecting your mother, grandmother, and aunt. It's the controlling men in your family who are behaving in a crazy way, and their behavior is abusive. It is abusive to control women, and it is abusive to treat you as crazy when all you are doing is reacting against being controlled."

"So what about my father's sister?" Isabella asked. "What about her? I've never met her. She cut herself off from the family before I was born, and Dad says that I'm crazy like her."

It took only a few answered questions for me to know that Isabella's father's sister was what I call a "Rebel Aunt." Discovering rebellious women is one of the exciting features of *Mother-Daughter History Maps*. They expose the women that families like to ostracize or pathologize because these rebel aunts are whistleblowers of the abuse women experience. In the past, whistleblowing women were locked away in attics or mental asylums, and still today in some male-dominated cultures, whistleblowing women are maimed or even killed. Rebellious women are courageous women who cannot buckle under being controlled or abused. They put their middle finger up in defiance against threats of being criticized, rejected from the family, or even killed, because they must fight for their rights.

It's a magical moment when a client discovers they're related to a rebellious woman. These kindred spirits make them feel less alone and less crazy. Someone else in the family also reacted to the family's abusive behavior, the emotional silencing and restrictive gender roles. And it's even more wonderful when a daughter realizes that her mother or grandmother were once rebels.

Rebellious women come in many shapes and sizes. Sometimes they come in the form of a mother's extraordinary courage to survive a horrific experience. Or a grandmother who had talents and intelligence beyond what her generation allowed her to realize. Isabella was, like her paternal aunt, her family's whistleblower. The so-called mental instability her father wanted me to cure her from was actually her healthy fight for freedom and emotional survival. Isabella did not want to repeat her mother's life and become emotionally silent like her, or critical like her grandmother. She didn't want her friends to take advantage of her need to be needed, as her mother's friends had.

But inside, Isabella's outward assertion was paper-thin. On the outside she appeared to be strong and tough, but inside she was insecure. She hated being the center of attention, even though she craved it. And even though she raged against being told what to do, on the inside, she didn't really know what she wanted. This was the work Isabella and I had to complete, so she didn't repeat the abuse and emotional silencing she had grown up with in her relationships.

To finish Isabella's map we had two more tasks to complete. First, we added arrows that told the story of who provided care and emotional support, and who received it. And second, we added zigzags to signify relationships that were troubled and abusive.

As you can see below, nearly all the arrows pointed away from Cynthia, showing how she provided all of the care and support in the family. Cynthia looked after her critical, demanding mother until she died, and she provided emotional support for her sister when her husband was violent. The only arrow pointing toward Cynthia came from Isabella, revealing the story of how Isabella had been given the role to emotionally support her mother. Isabella said that she tried to encourage her mother to stand up for herself against her husband, and to say no when people were too demanding of her, but her mother didn't listen. With tears in her eyes,

Isabella said, "I feel like my relationship with my mom is a one-way street. I give her emotional support, and she guilt-trips me for causing trouble and making her exhausted."

This was an example of the river of nurturing flowing backwards up the generations, which I explained in Chapter 4, rather than down the generations from mother to daughter, as it should flow at Isabella's age. Isabella's generational family showed how this dynamic is indicative of families where women are emotionally neglected, and the daughter, often the elder or eldest daughter, is given the role of being the mother's emotional caregiver. But Isabella was still young. She needed the emotional caring between her mother and her to flow downward, from her mother to herself. And as she grew up and became an adult, she needed her relationship with her mother to become more mutually supportive, as I explained in Chapter 4.

But if Isabella and her mother, and father, didn't change the narrative in their family about how women were emotionally neglected, it was going to be impossible for Isabella and her mother to create a mutually supportive, woman-to-woman relationship in the future. At sixteen, Isabella was already acting like a grown-up. She was the one who questioned when things were wrong and worried about what her mother needed, without receiving the same attention and care in return. And I could predict with great certainty that if Isabella didn't learn how to claim what she needed and speak her own emotional truth, she would inherit her mother's emotional starvation, and the sad history would repeat itself—Isabella's future daughter would be angry with Isabella for not being able to teach her how to be heard.

We then added the zigzags, revealing the many troubled and abusive relationships in Isabella's generational family. Isabella's relationship with her father and mother was troubled and abusive. Cynthia had a troubled and abusive relationship with her mother, father, and husband. All the men were abusive toward their wives. And all these zigzags revealed that in this family no one felt heard, understood, emotionally supported, or loved.

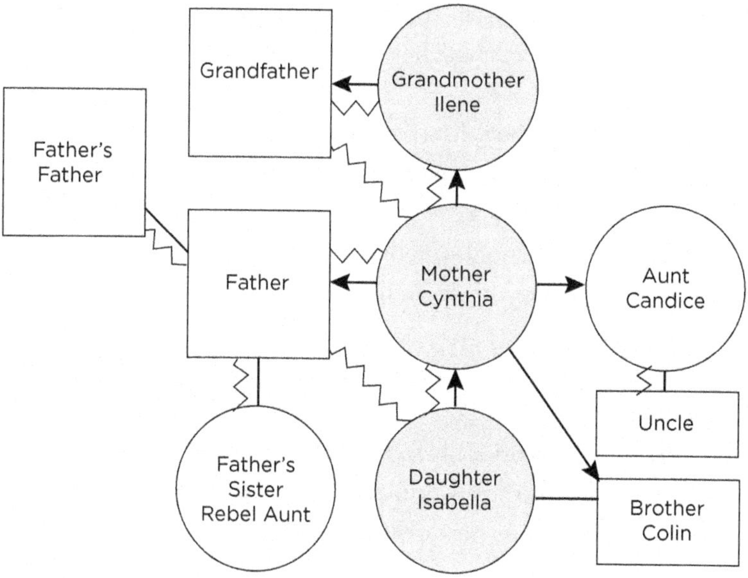

The final task in the *Mother-Daughter History Mapping* exercise was to create a roadmap for change for Isabella. On a separate piece of paper, I wrote the following themes in her mother-daughter history:

- Women have no needs voice. They listen and accommodate rather than speak and advocate for themselves.
- Women are invisible, emotionally neglected, and emotionally starved.
- Women are selfless caregivers.
- Fathers and husbands are selfish, emotionally abusive, or violent.
- Daughters provide the emotional support their mother cannot give them and that they aren't receiving from their family, friends, and husband.
- Daughters aren't heard, understood, or emotionally supported by their mother, which harms a daughter's ability to feel loved and worthy of being loved.

- Women have learned to cope with their emotional emptiness by controlling what they eat and how much they weigh.

Then, using the above list, I wrote the following roadmap of goals that Isabella needed to work on for her healing and empowerment:

- Identify what she needs emotionally.
- Feel comfortable with speaking what she feels, needs, thinks, and wants.
- Walk away from relationships where her voice is not inquired after and honored.
- Learn how to emotionally feed herself.
- Believe in her intrinsic worth as a human being and that her worth is not dependent on how well she cares for others.

Isabella took her map home with her because she was excited about what she had learned and she wanted to tell her parents about it. Experience warned me that this wouldn't be well received by her father. But I was wrong. What happened next was a miracle.

The next week her father came with Isabella to her session. He was a tall, thickset man with an imposing, even dominating feel about him. My first thought was that he had come because he was angry about my session with Isabella. I was mistaken! As soon as he walked into my office, he extended his hand and thanked me for Isabella's *Mother-Daughter History Map*. Isabella had made him see that he, and all the men in the family, were abusive, and felt far too entitled to control everyone. He told me how he had suffered under his father's extreme need for control, and he was shocked and deeply sorry that he had turned into his father. He told me that the *Mother-Daughter History Map* had made him realize that he was to blame for Isabella's rebellious behavior.

Isabella looked like a different girl sitting next to her father. Her makeup was more subtle and her long brown hair was tied up in a ponytail, no longer hanging loose over her face. It was wonderful to see how much her father's affirmation had both emboldened her and softened her. Gone was the angry, silent girl I had met only a few sessions ago. In her place was an emotionally open, talkative girl.

Over time, Isabella's relationship with her parents improved. Her parents learned to listen to her, and consequently, she didn't need to be rebellious anymore to be noticed. Isabella and her mom learned how to speak what they needed, and to feel comfortable with being heard. And her father reconnected with his long-lost sister.

This exercise saved Isabella from being estranged from her family. It taught them the valuable lesson that if you silence someone's emotional truth and stop them from claiming their autonomy, you lose them. Isabella's father had lost his sister years ago because she wasn't allowed to make her own decisions. If he hadn't taken her *Mother-Daughter History Map* to heart, he would have lost his daughter as well.

I don't always get miraculous results with families as I did with Isabella's family, because not every family is willing to have their hidden truths and secrets exposed. Mapping a woman's mother-daughter history is a powerful exercise that is a little like completing a jigsaw puzzle. We start by laying out all the pieces of information we know, and then we fit the pieces together to create a picture of what it means to be female in her multigenerational family. Inevitably, some of the information won't fit into the overall picture. Stories can sometimes not make sense, and information gaps emerge. When this happens, it's likely that a family secret is being withheld. Secrets make themselves known through gaps in knowledge, unanswered questions, and topics that are surrounded by an aura of anger, fear, and shame.

Every time I draw out a client's *Mother-Daughter History Map*, I'm blown away about how this exercise emboldens women to reveal truths they have never told. I see the healing women receive when their secrets are witnessed and recorded. They no longer have to carry the shame of how they've been mistreated. Through their *Mother-Daughter History Map*, they return the shame of the abuse back to the perpetrator where it belongs.

I find that when women gather in *Women's Power Circles* (see Chapter 9) and map their mother-daughter history together, this exercise becomes even more transformational. When women listen to the themes and stories in each other's maps, they learn how similar women's lives are when we uncover women's generational experiences of emotional silence and neglect. Women recognize that they are not alone, and that we all come from families that have muzzled women's voices, denied their truths, and ignored their needs. We all harbor stories of shamed women who had a child out of wedlock, of the deadly consequences of illegal abortions, of rape and genital mutilation, of being wed too young and without choice, of being undereducated, and of losing your family because in your culture, wives are expected to join the husband's family.

Mother-Daughter History Maps make the political personal. They show how women have been harmed by generations of male domination and misogyny, and it's essential that we understand this, so the harm isn't repeated today and in future generations. In the next chapter, have a go at mapping your own mother-daughter history.

ISABELLA'S MOTHER-DAUGHTER HISTORY MAP

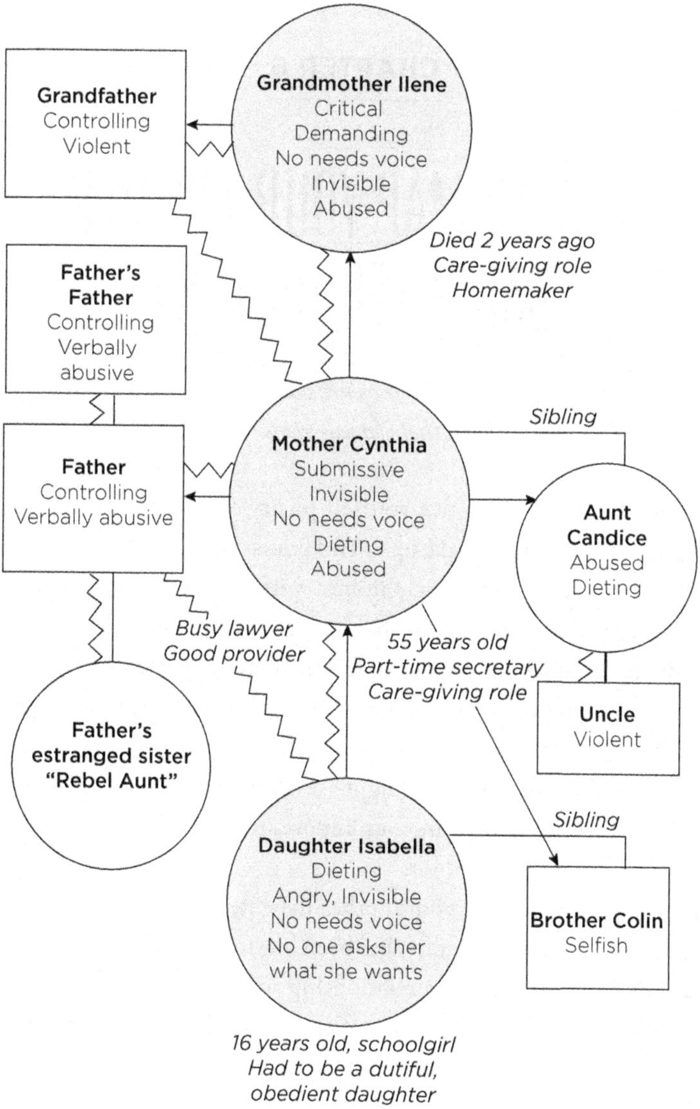

CHAPTER 6

HOW TO MAP YOUR MOTHER-DAUGHTER HISTORY

Women discover who they are when they learn about their female roots.

I SUGGEST THAT YOU give yourself plenty of time to complete this exercise, because it can take up to two hours. And because this exercise asks that you are completely honest with yourself, and to tell hard truths about your life and your family relationships, it's important that you do this exercise in a comfortable, safe space, and when you're feeling happy and content. It isn't a good idea to do this exercise just after you've had an argument with your mother, father, or other family members, because heightened emotions might skew your results.

Before we begin, here are four important ground rules.

1. You are the daughter in your mother-daughter history map.
To get a full picture of what life has been like for the three key women in your family, as well as your relationship with your mother, and your mother's relationship with her mother, you need to be the daughter in your *Mother-Daughter History Map*.

2. This is a map of what *you* feel and what *you* think happened.
Mapping your mother-daughter history is a very personal exercise. It's a record of what you know happened in your life, and what you think hap-

pened in the lives of your mother and grandmother. It's a record of how you feel about your relationship with your mother, and your perceptions of your mother and grandmother's relationship, along with how you feel about how your father and grandfather treated your mother and grandmother.

It's important that you tell the truth when you map your history. It can be tempting to ignore something, or deny that something happened, but this will only lessen the power of this exercise. Your truth includes what you feel, think, and know about yourself, and what you feel, think, and know about the lives of your parents, grandparents, and other relatives.

Your truth also includes what you suspect. Hunches and gut feelings are an important part of this exercise because they can help uncover beliefs, behavioral patterns, and family secrets that no one talks about. When mapping your mother-daughter history, write down what you suspect is true about your mother's and grandmother's lives. Write down what you think is the honest truth when your mother gives a false smile or says she's fine, when you know she isn't.

3. This map is a record of your life now.

When recording an issue that has changed in your life, it's important to first record how it is for you now, and then add a short note about how it used to be before. For example, today I would record that I don't feel responsible if someone is angry with me because I'm not doing what he or she wants me to do. And then I would add that in the past I did feel responsible for other people's happiness. As a child I was taught to feel super-responsible for other people's needs and feelings, especially my mother's, and the women in my family are socialized to take responsibility for other people's needs and happiness, not their own.

4. Map with a trusted friend.

Mapping your mother-daughter history is an emotionally demanding exercise that is best done with a supportive friend or sister, or your mother, if you have an emotionally open relationship with her. Mapping in pairs enables you to talk through your answers and hunches. It can give you greater clarity about your thoughts and perceptions. It is healing to have your story witnessed by someone you trust.

It's also very revealing when a mother and daughter, or sisters, map their respective maps and then compare their results. It's enlightening to see the similar themes and issues and how your perceptions and experiences differ.

Make sure you choose the right person with whom to map your mother-daughter history. Choose someone you trust with your story and who will keep it confidential. Choose someone who will honor what you say and be gentle with your feelings and not judge you or be critical of you. Choose someone who is insightful, and who is not afraid to ask the hard questions, to question the status quo, and to dig below the surface to uncover beliefs and norms that the women in your family have lived with for generations.

8-Step Mother-Daughter History Mapping Instructions

You will need:

One large piece of paper
Sharp pencil and eraser
Highlighter

Step 1: Copy the template onto a large piece of paper.
(The template is at the end of this chapter.)

Step 2: Write in the names as follows.
Circles represent females, and squares represent males, as in traditional genograms.

Start with the three central women and write your name in the "Daughter" circle, your mother's name in the "Mother" circle, and your grandmother's (your mother's mother) in the "Grandmother" circle.

Write the names of the men in the squares on the left. Write your father's name in the "Father" square, your grandfather's name (mother's father) in the "Grandfather" square, and your husband, partner, or boyfriend in the "Husband/partner" square. If you have an ex-husband, and other significant boyfriends, add more squares to this line of your map. And if your mother or grandmother had ex-husbands or significant boyfriends, add them as well, next to your father or grandfather.

Add in the names of your father's mother and father in the "Father's Father" square and "Father's Mother" circle.

Add in the names of your parents-in-law, if you have them, in the "Father-in-law" square and "Mother-in-law" circle.

Fill in the names of your siblings and the names of your mother's siblings on the right-hand side of the page. (For the purpose of this exercise, we only focus on yours and your mother's siblings.) Start with female siblings in circles, and then add male siblings in squares. Birth order doesn't matter all that much in mother-daughter history maps, except for the role of being the elder/eldest daughter.

Mark all elder/eldest daughters with a big "E-D," because it highlights who might have been expected to meet their mother's unspoken feelings and denied emotional needs.

Don't worry if you don't know everyone's name. Record the names you know, and for those you don't know, record them as a question mark in their circle or square.

Add any children you have at the bottom of the page, below your circle. Record a daughter in a circle and a son in a square.

This template is a guide, and I encourage you to be innovative, because all families are different. Fit your family around the three central women. Add whomever you think is significant. If your history includes stepfathers, stepmothers, and stepbrothers/sisters, add them in. If you are adopted, next to your adopted mother and father add your biological mother and father in their circle and square, even if you don't know who they are. It's important to give your biological mother a place on your map because she is part of your story. You spent the first nine months of your life in her body, soaking in her emotions and beliefs, which current research suggests has an important influence on who we are and how we react to things.

Step 3: Let's start with you, your mother, and your grandmother.

It's important to separate out the facts about who we are, and who our mother and grandmother is, or was, and the emotional reality we each live in.

Facts include: the age someone is, the age someone died, their level of education, occupation, significant life events, and what gender roles they had to comply with, like being a stay-at-home mother and caregiver.

Emotional Reality includes: whether we feel heard, and whether we believe our mother and grandmother were heard and emotionally supported. It includes whether we know what we need emotionally, or diet a lot, suffer from an eating disorder or other mental or emotional issues like depression or anxiety, and if we were physically or sexually abused.

Following are two lists of questions. The first list asks you to record the *facts* about you, your mother, and your grandmother. Record the answers around the *outside* of your own, your mother's, and your grandmother's circles.

The second list asks you to record your own *emotional reality*, what you believe is (or was, if your mother and grandmother have died) your mother's and grandmother's emotional realities. Record these answers *inside* your own and inside your mother's and grandmother's circles.

Record all answers as keywords or short phrases to conserve space. Use words that remind you of what you mean.

Don't worry if you don't know the answer to a particular question. When you don't know the answer to a question, write a short summary of the question along with a question mark (?) on your map. Question marks are important! They are an integral part of your family's emotional reality, because they record what isn't known about someone, who is invisible, and what is secret.

Fact questions: Record the answers as keywords or short phrases around the *outside* of your own, your mother's, and your grandmother's circles.

1. How old are you? And how old is your mother and grandmother? If your mother and/or grandmother have died, when did they die and how old were they?
2. What is your level of education? And what was your mother's and grandmother's level of education? Record if you, or your mother and grandmother, weren't allowed to realize their educational or occupational ambitions.
3. What is your occupation? And what was your mother's and grandmother's occupation? "Stay-at-home mother" is of course an occupation.
4. What gender roles are/were you, and your mother and grandmother, expected to comply with? Gender roles include whatever your family and culture believe is a woman's role. For example, being a caregiver, a stay-at-home mother, a supermom, self-sacrificing, arranged marriage, no access to contraception or legal abortion, and prioritizing of men's needs and lives.

Emotional Reality questions: Record the answer as keywords or short phrases *inside* of your own, your mother's, and your grandmother's circles. Remember to record questions that you don't know the answer to with a question mark. And it doesn't matter if your mother or grandmother disagrees with your answers, because this is a record of what *you* think is true.

1. How do you voice what you need? And how does or did your mother and grandmother voice what they need? If any of you don't/didn't voice what you need, write "no needs voice" in your respective circle.
2. How are your emotional needs inquired after and heard? And how are, or were, your mother's and grandmother's emotional needs inquired after and heard? If any of your emotional needs aren't inquired after or heard, write "emotionally neglected" in your respective circle.
3. What emotional struggles do you, your mother, and grandmother suffer from? Emotional struggles include issues like eating disorders, depression, and anxiety, as well as being excessively caring and neglecting

yourself, being submissive and unable to advocate for yourself, being critical and demanding, and being emotionally manipulative.

4. What strengths and resilience do you have, and your mother and grandmother have or had? This includes positive changes that you, your mother, and grandmother have made to emotionally empower yourselves and challenge and change disempowering gender roles.

Step 4: Now for your siblings and your mother's siblings.

For the purpose of this mapping exercise, we'll only focus on your siblings and your mother's siblings.

Let's start with the female siblings.

Fact questions for your, and your mother's, female siblings: Record the answers as keywords or short phrases around the *outside* of their circles.

1. What is, or was, their occupation? Were any female siblings not able to realize their dreams?
2. What gender roles did they comply with?

Emotional Reality questions for your, and your mother's, female siblings: Record the answers as keywords or short-phrase answers *inside* their circles.

1. How do, or did, they voice what they need? Record "no needs voice" if they are emotionally silent.
2. How do, or did, they meet their emotional needs? Record "emotionally neglected" if they were emotionally neglected.
3. What emotional struggles do, or did, they suffer from?
4. What were/are their strengths and resilience? Are there any "rebel aunts" who have rejected the family's role expectations?

Questions for your and your mother's male siblings: Record the answers as keywords and short phrases *inside* their squares.

1. How do, or did, they treat their sisters when they were young? Were they kind and caring or harsh and abusive?

2. When young, were the boys expected to help out at home or were they free to do whatever they wanted?
3. When young, did the boys have the same educational opportunities as their sisters, or were the boys given more opportunities and resources?
4. How emotionally supportive are your brothers and your mother's brothers today? Do they help with caring for sick or elderly family members? Do they inquire after what their wives and daughters need and emotionally support their dreams and goals? If not, record "emotionally neglecting" in their squares.

Step 5: Let's look at how loving and emotionally supportive the men are in your family.

The following questions explore how the three primary men in your family—your boyfriend, partner, or husband, father, and grandfather, treat women, and how their behavior affects or affected you, your mother, and grandmother.

Again, there are *Fact* questions to answer as keywords or short phrases around the *outside* of the men's squares, and *Emotional Reality* questions to answer as keywords and short phrases *inside* their squares.

Fact questions:

1. What gender roles do, or did, your husband, partner, or boyfriend, father, and grandfather comply with? For example, were they a good provider, valued for their physical strength, not allowed to cry or express their emotions? Or, did they believe in doing their share of domestic work like cooking, cleaning, and childrearing?
2. What jobs and level of education do, or did, your husband, partner, or boyfriend, father, and grandfather have?

Emotional Reality questions:

1. Do you feel heard by your husband, partner, or boyfriend? Is what you want inquired after and honored with the same degree of importance as what he wants? If not, record "emotionally neglecting." And

does, or did, your father and grandfather listen to your mother and grandmother? If not, record "emotionally neglecting."

2. Are any of these men selfish, critical, a bully, violent, alcoholic, sexually or emotionally abusive, unfaithful, emotionally manipulative, or emotionally silent?
3. Do any of these men favor sons over daughters?

Step 6: Let's look at your father's parents and your parents-in-law (if you have any).

Record your answers as keywords or short phrases to the *Fact* questions around the *outside* of their respective circle or square, and the *Emotional Reality* questions on the *inside* of their circle or square.

I have separated out the following questions by gender to give a clearer picture of your paternal grandmother's, and mother-in-law's, emotional realities, and the role the men play in creating them.

Fact questions for your father's mother and your mother-in-law.

1. What is their age, or if they have died, how old were they when they died?
2. What was their level of education? Record if they did not realize their educational or career goals.
3. What is, or was, their occupation? Were they a stay-at-home mother?
4. What gender roles were they expected to comply with? For example, being a caregiver, a stay-at-home mother, a supermom, self-sacrificing, arranged marriage, no access to contraception or legal abortion, and prioritizing of men's need and lives.

Emotional Reality for your father's mother and your mother-in-law.

1. Do they voice what they need? If not, record "no needs voice."
2. How is what they need emotionally inquired after and heard by their families? If it's not, record "emotionally neglected."
3. What emotional struggles do, or did, they suffer from? For example, eating disorders, depression, and anxiety, as well as behaviors like

excessive caregiving and being neglectful of themselves, being submissive and not knowing how to advocate for themselves, being critical and demanding, and emotionally manipulative.

4. What strengths and resilience do, or did, they have? What positive changes have they facilitated in their lives? What disempowering gender roles have they challenged and changed?
5. How does your father's mother treat your mother, her daughter-in-law, and how does your mother-in-law treat you? Are they supportive and complimentary, or critical and demanding? Do they treat you and your mother as people in your own right, or do they believe it is your role and your mother's role to spend your lives taking care of your husband and family? And do they expect you and your mother to take care of them and meet their needs?

Fact questions for your father's father and your father-in-law.

1. What gender roles do, or did, they comply with? For example, were they a good provider, valued for their physical strength, not allowed to cry or express their emotions, or did they believe in doing their share of domestic work like cooking, cleaning, and childrearing?
2. What jobs and level of education do, or did, they have?

Emotional Reality questions for your father's father and your father-in-law:

1. How do, or did, they treat their wives? For example, do, or did they listen, or were they dismissive? Are, or were they loving or abusive? Do, or did they appreciate what their wives provided or were/are they critical of her? If dismissive and critical, record "emotionally neglecting."
2. Are, or were any of these men violent, alcoholic, sexually or emotionally abusive, unfaithful, emotionally manipulative, or emotionally silent?
3. Do, or did they favor sons over daughters?
4. How does/did your father's father treat your mother, his daughter-in-law, and how does/did your father-in-law treat you? Does your

father-in-law listen to you and respect your feelings and needs, and does your mother's father-in-law listen to her and respect her feelings and needs? And does your father-in-law treat you as if you are in service to your husband and children, and does your mother's father-in-law treat your mother in the same way?

Step 7: Now let's map out relationships.

The focus of this step is to describe the relationships in your family in terms of who does all the emotional caring. I use four symbols to describe family relationships.

An arrow (→) describes the direction in which the emotional care flows within a relationship. Though women do a great deal of the physical caregiving, in mother-daughter history maps, an arrow describes the emotional caregiving women provide, and who is the giver and the recipient.

A zigzag (⁄\⁄) describes a troubled or conflicted relationship. For example, a relationship where there is severe conflict or estrangement, or one suffering from emotionally manipulative or passive-aggressive behavior.

A double vertical line (**||**) describes a relationship that has ended in separation or divorce.

A double horizontal line (=) describes a strong, mutually supportive, loving relationship.

Let's draw arrows.

1. Draw an arrow between you and your mother, pointing *from* whom provides most of the emotional caregiving *to* the person receiving it. If the listening and emotional support that is being given and received in your relationship is mutual, draw two arrows, one pointing from you to your mother and the other from your mother to you.
2. Draw an arrow between your mother and grandmother, pointing from whom provides most of the emotional caregiving to the person receiving it. If you believe that your mother and grandmother have a mutually supportive relationship, draw an arrowhead at each end.

If the caregiving has changed between your mother and grandmother, draw an arrow that reflects their relationship now.

3. Draw an arrow between you and your siblings to indicate who does most of the emotional caregiving. If any relationship with a sibling is mutually supportive, draw two arrowheads.
4. Draw an arrow between your mother and her siblings to indicate who does most of the emotional caregiving. Again, if any relationships are mutually supportive, draw two arrowheads.
5. Draw arrows between your mother and her husband, and your mother and her father, pointing from the person who does, or did, most of the emotional caregiving to the one who does, or did, most of the receiving.
6. Draw an arrow between your grandmother and her husband, pointing from the person who does, or did, most of the emotional caregiving to the one who does, or did, most of the receiving.
7. And finally, draw arrows between you and your husband, partner, or boyfriend, and you and your father, pointing from who does most of the emotional caregiving to the one who does, or did, most of the receiving. If any of these relationships are mutually supportive, draw an arrowhead at each end.

Let's draw zigzags.

1. Draw a zigzag between you and your mother, or your mother and your grandmother, if these relationships are conflicted, angry, estranged, or display emotionally manipulative or passive-aggressive behavior.
2. Draw a zigzag between you and your siblings, and your mother and her siblings, if any of these relationships are conflicted, angry, estranged, or display emotionally manipulative or passive-aggressive behavior.
3. Draw a zigzag between you and your husband, partner, or boyfriend, your mother and her husband, and your grandmother and her husband, if any of these relationships are conflicted or angry.

4. Draw a zigzag between you and your father, and your mother and her father, if any of these relationships are conflicted or angry.
5. Draw a zigzag between your mother and her in-laws, and you and your in-laws, if you have any, if any of these relationships are conflicted or angry.

Let's draw double vertical lines.

- Draw a double vertical line between any relationship that has ended in separation or divorce.

And finally, let's draw double horizontal lines

- Draw a double horizontal line between any relationship that is loving, emotionally nurturing, empowering of women's rights and equality, and mutually supportive.

Step 8: You are nearly done! Let's create a roadmap for change.

This last stage can be emotionally challenging at first, but as you go through it, you will feel stronger in your resolve to claim what you need emotionally and create the generational change you deserve.

With a highlighter, highlight:

1. The women who are emotionally neglected, emotionally starved, have no needs voice, and are invisible. Notice how these themes repeat themselves generation after generation.
2. *Emotional Reality* themes where women are behaving in a critical, emotionally manipulative, and controlling way, and struggle with emotional struggles like eating disorders and depression. Notice how these themes correlate with the emotional neglect in number one, and how they repeat themselves generation after generation.
3. Themes where women's goals and dreams were not realized.
4. The women who have been abused. Again notice how this theme repeats itself generation after generation.

5. The men who emotionally neglect women and favor sons over daughters. And notice how this theme repeats itself generation after generation.
6. Arrows where the emotional caregiving flows backwards, from the daughter to mother, rather than forward from the mother to daughter. Notice how this theme correlates with the emotional neglect and emotionally manipulative behavior themes.

At the top left corner of the page, list the above themes that you have highlighted. For example:

- Women don't know what they need.
- Women's needs are not inquired after or understood.
- Women focus more on what men need, rather than what they need.
- Men are emotionally absent.
- Emotional caring flows backwards from daughters to mothers.
- Women are expected to care, fit in, and accommodate.
- Women are invisible.

Draw a line above you, and also your mother if you and your mother are joining forces to change your female legacy. This line is your *line of change*, which represents that from now on, things are going to be different for you (and your mom), and future generations of women in your family.

At the top right corner of the page, using the list on the left, make a to-do list that reflects what needs to be changed. For example:

1. Women need to identify and value what they need.
2. Women's feelings, needs, and thoughts must be inquired after and honored.
3. Women's worth is not defined by their caregiving role.
4. Women can advocate for themselves.

These themes are your "Roadmap for Creating Generational Change." They are a guide to creating an emotional environment where you, your mom, and your daughter if you have one, are heard, understood, emotionally supported, and free to make your own decisions. Read the remaining chapters for guidance on how to claim your emotional needs, change negative generational patterns, and strengthen all your female relationships.

Well done! You have accomplished the brave emotional work of mapping your mother-daughter history. This work isn't easy. Seeing the bold truth of your own life and the emotional reality you grew up in is not for the fainthearted. But it is lifesaving! One woman told me after we mapped her mother-daughter history, she felt released from the weight of responsibilities that were not hers. Another told me how shocked and deeply saddened she felt when she discovered how unloved her mother and grandmother had been. Recognizing this emotional truth helped her see how she, too, was tolerating relationships in which she was unloved and invisible. Two years later, she emailed me her wedding photos, thanking me for waking her up, because this information had helped her find a man who saw her and loved her. It was heartwarming to see how radiant she looked on her wedding day.

I applaud this woman's courage, and all women who dare to wake up and make a stand against generations of misogynistic tradition. And because of their courage, their daughters and sons will inherit a different legacy—one where women are heard, emotionally supported, loved, and respected. Surely all women deserve to live in this emotional reality.

MOTHER-DAUGHTER HISTORY MAP TEMPLATE

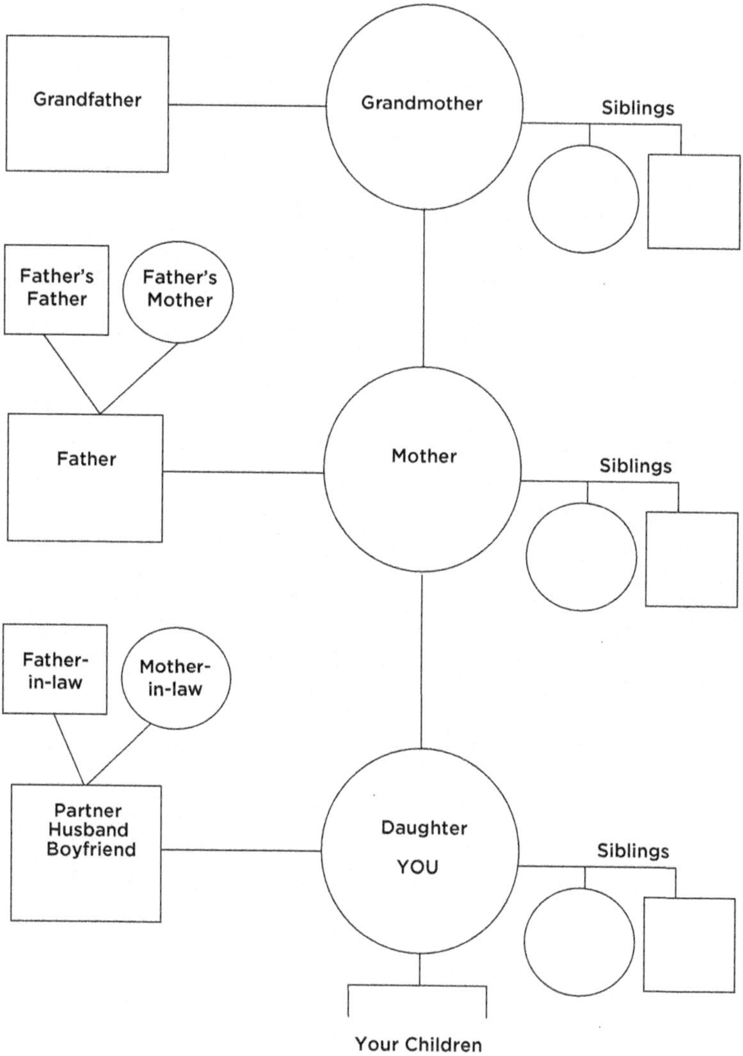

PART THREE

USING THE PUZZLE FOR CHANGE

CHAPTER 7

SPEAKING YOUR TRUTH, CLAIMING YOUR EMOTIONAL NEEDS, AND BEING TAKEN SERIOUSLY

A woman who knows what she needs cannot be controlled.

SHAMING WOMEN FOR having needs of their own has been a powerful, centuries-old patriarchal strategy that co-opts women into complying with their own inequality. As I wrote in *The Silent Female Scream*, women "cannot thrive, or be equal or empowered, if we do not need."[1] Client after client, I hear how women have learned to normalize being emotionally silenced, and how infrequently they notice that their emotional silence makes them invisible and unequal in their relationships, and at work. In *Mother-Daughter History Maps*, I see how, generation after generation, women learn to believe that needing is bad, that not being heard or emotionally supported is a "woman's lot," as my grandmother used to say, and how mothers teach their daughters how to disregard their needs. I see how mothers and daughters tune into what their father, husband, children, and friends need, because they believe it is their duty to advocate for other people's needs, while their needs come a poor second, if they even address them at all. And I see these themes so consistently, I have yet to meet a woman who hasn't in some way learned to silence herself.

Thankfully, change is happening! I am seeing women of all ages and from different countries and cultures waking up to the realization that "needing" makes them human. That needing is central to their equality, and their ability to have agency over their lives. Women are connecting the dots between their inherited emotional silence and their invisibility in relationships, their inequality at work, their symptoms of emotional starvation, their drive for perfection, their mother-daughter conflict, and their struggles with depression, anxiety, and eating disorders.

I worked with Miriam, the mother, and Abigail, the daughter, through Skype, because they were from Sweden. Their story was a compelling one, because outwardly this feminist mother-daughter couple didn't appear to have any problems with knowing what they wanted and needed. Miriam and Abigail came from a generational family in which the women achieved career goals and financial independence well ahead of their time. Miriam's grandmother ran a successful shop, selling sewing supplies and homemade jams. Miriam's mother was a doctor, the only female in her graduating class. Miriam was a much sought-after knee surgeon and Abigail a high-achieving senior in high school, with an offer to study history at Oxford University. Miriam's father and grandfather were loving men who encouraged their wives' and daughters' career goals. And Pontus, Miriam's husband and Abigail's father, was a feminist, who believed in emotionally supporting his wife and daughter. Yet, underneath all this high achievement and apparent gender equality, Miriam and Abigail were emotionally mute. Their ability to advocate for themselves at work and school wasn't transferring into their personal relationships.

Miriam and Abigail's mother-daughter story shows how women's emotional entitlement to have their needs and voices matter in their relationships lags behind the advances women have made over the last generations. Just as how "trickle-down economics" doesn't work, having women's human rights enshrined in law doesn't necessarily "trickle down" to raise women's individual entitlement to speak and be heard. And marrying an emotionally in-tune man, though necessary for a relationship in which a woman feels heard and emotionally supported, doesn't automatically make her know what she needs, or enable her to be emotionally literate. We all need to individually, and collectively, claim our entitlement to need and to challenge the beliefs and stereotypes that silence us from expressing our needs.

Miriam called me for an appointment for her and Abigail because she was concerned about how Abigail had changed over the last six months, from being a happy and outgoing person to being depressed and withdrawn. Pontus also wanted to join in the sessions; he was worried about his daughter and he wanted to know what he could do to help her.

As their first session began, I saw Miriam, Abigail, and Pontus sitting crammed up together in front of their computer. Miriam was dressed in a blue and white-striped tee shirt, and my first impression of her was that she was a jolly person who liked to have fun. I noticed how much alike Abigail and her mom were. Abigail's brown hair was longer than her mother's, whose hair was cut short. Abigail was also wearing a blue tee shirt, though whether her choice to wear the same color as her mother was intentional, I couldn't tell. Pontus was a tall, thin man with blond hair who also, at first impression, looked like a fun-loving person.

Miriam was the first to speak. She said, "We are really hoping you can make sense of why Abigail has become withdrawn and angry." As she glanced at Pontus and Abigail she continued. "We're very worried about Abigail and we want the old Abigail back."

As I listened to Miriam, Abigail, and Pontus talk about their family life, it sounded picture perfect. Abigail described her father as "the gentlest man ever," and she loved having her own special outings with each parent. Abigail and Pontus went fishing most Sunday mornings during the summer months, and Miriam and Abigail had their weekly yoga class, followed by coffee at a local coffee shop. But something wasn't working for Abigail, and I was eager to dig below the surface and discover what was making her feel depressed.

Mapping Miriam's Mother-Daughter History

I decided to map Miriam's mother-daughter history, rather than Abigail's, because I wanted to understand Miriam's inherited emotional legacy, to understand what themes had been passed down to her from her grandmother. Normally I map a client's mother-daughter history in private, but since this family seemed so emotionally close, I felt it would be beneficial for Abigail and Pontus to witness the mapping of Miriam's female history.

In Miriam's *Mother-Daughter History Map* we saw how her parents and grandparents, though sadly dead, were loving people. Miriam's mother and grandmother were strong, determined women, and her father and grandfather loved their wives. But as we explored how the Culture of Female Service had defined Miriam's mother's and grandmother's lives, clues about what was upsetting Abigail started to reveal themselves. Though Miriam and her mother had benefited from the women's movement and achieved a voice and identity outside their domestic duties, when it came to voicing what they needed emotionally as mothers, they were both silent. The power they had gained as doctors, to have their wishes taken seriously, hadn't influenced how they mothered. As mothers, they had repeated the centuries-old tradition of selfless mothering, which had caused them to be emotionally mute in their relationships with their husbands and daughters.

When I asked Miriam to describe her mother, her face brightened. She described how clever her mother had been, and how everyone loved her. How she had the kind of house to which neighborhood children flocked. Even though she was busy, she always had homemade cookies and a kind word for everyone. Yet, when I asked Miriam to describe who her mom was as a woman and not as a wife, mother, or doctor, and what her mother needed emotionally, Miriam fell silent, and her expression told me she didn't know how to answer this question.

The silence lengthened, until she said, "I feel so sad that I never got to know Mom as a person. In our family she was always Mom. Everyone loved her as Mom, and it never occurred to me to see her in any other way. And I think Mom didn't know that she existed outside of her caregiving roles. She loved Dad, and she loved taking care of everyone."

I then asked Miriam to list what emotional needs she had in her relationship with her husband and daughter, and Miriam responded with the same blank look I see on many of my clients' faces. After a moment of awkward silence, Miriam did what many emotionally mute clients do; she skillfully circumvented the question by talking about what she thought her daughter needed.

Miriam was the quintessential superwoman. She juggled a demanding job and family responsibilities with such finesse, I felt fatigue at listening to all she did. And because Pontus anticipated what Miriam needed, Miriam was spared from experiencing the horrible emotional consequences of her self-neglecting behavior. Unlike other women, Miriam didn't have to scream to be heard, or become emotionally manipulative to have her needs meet. Her husband was a master mind reader, who knew Miriam better than she knew herself. But this dynamic had been causing conflict between Miriam and Abigail, and for some time.

Miriam and Abigail's relationship story reveals the paradox of how women who excel at responding to other people's needs can struggle to listen to and understand their own needs, and their daughter's. From when Abigail was a young girl, Miriam had struggled to really listen to and understand Abigail's point of view, especially when it was different from hers. Now that Abigail was growing up and leaving home to go to Oxford, Miriam's inability to navigate her daughter's emotional reality was starting to cause problems. Abigail had become increasingly frustrated with her mother's inability to really understand her, and she also hated that she didn't know what her mother was thinking. The only way Abigail knew what was going on in her mother's mind was through her father's ability to accurately interpret his wife's emotional state.

I've told Miriam and Abigail's mother-daughter story because their relationship struggles, and Abigail's depression, which turned out to be made more complex by the problems she was having with her girlfriends, tells the story of how even women who seem to have it all are waking up to their internalized, and inherited, emotional silence.

As the following equation shows, for mothers and daughters, being heard and understood is inextricably linked to feeling loved, which explains how emotional silencing creates conflict between mothers and daughters. When a mother or daughter doesn't know how to voice what she's feeling, thinking, and needing, her ability to communicate the love that is hard-wired into their relationship is harmed. And without this conversation, mothers and daughters are in danger of feeling unloved.

Being Heard + Being Understood = Feeling Loved.[2]

Another dynamic in Miriam's mother-daughter history revealed how her relationship with her mother hadn't evolved into a mutually supportive relationship, as it should have. Miriam's mother had been content meeting her daughter's needs, and everyone else's needs, throughout her life. And as an adult, Miriam had been happy for her mother to continue mothering her. It wasn't until our therapy sessions that Miriam became aware of how this dynamic—continuing to rely on her mother and her mother's willingness to allow the dependence—had stopped her from knowing her mother as a person. And now Miriam was on track to repeat this dynamic with Abigail, which was what Abigail was fighting against. Abigail's depression was a reaction against, a rebelling from, never growing up to be a person in her own right in her relationship with her mother, not wanting to inherit her mother's and grandmother's emotional silence, and not wanting to have her life defined by how well she herself takes care of people.

Women Silencing Each Other

As Abigail looked at her mother's *Mother-Daughter History Map*, she pointed to how emotional silence had been passed down the generations, and she said, "I don't want this! I couldn't tell you what was wrong until now, but here it is. I do not want to grow up relying on you, or Dad, or my future husband, or other people, to say what I need. I want to say it for myself."

Facing her mom, she continued speaking. "I feel terribly guilty when I get angry when you don't put yourself first, and when you expect Dad to mind-read your needs. It makes me feel that I am being ungrateful if I say that I resent the way you are, Mom. But the truth is I don't want this for me, or for you. I love you and I don't want to hurt you, but I want you to be you, and me to be me, as well as being a mother and daughter."

Miriam and Pontus looked both shocked and relieved as their daughter shared what was wrong. Miriam was close to tears, and I could see that there were many thoughts and emotions swirling around in her mind. Pontus was the first to speak. Turning to Miriam, he said in a quiet voice, "You know, I sometimes feel that you forget I'm here, that I'm just as responsible as you for taking care of our family."

Miriam nodded, and as she turned to him she said in a shaky voice, "I know I need to change this. Not just with you, but in all my relationships. I know at work I'm too nice. I don't advocate for myself as much as I should, and I end up shouldering responsibility that isn't mine to shoulder."

At this point the conversation turned to Abigail's friends, a clique of girls who hung out together at school and on the weekends. Miriam knew and liked Abigail's friends and was glad her daughter was part of this group, but as we were about to discover, Abigail's depression was, in part, being caused by some nasty dynamics in this group.

Having already inherited her mother and grandmother's role of being a caretaker, her friends turned to Abigail whenever they had a problem. But whenever Abigail needed a listening ear, they didn't return the favor. Her friends expected Abigail to be caring and accommodating, and up until about six months before, Abigail had been okay with playing this role. But she was changing, growing into her power, and she wanted her friends to start listening to her.

Abigail had been keeping her feelings to herself because she wasn't sure how to tell her friends that she didn't like how little they listened to her. When she desperately wanted to see a particular movie, she decided it was time to be courageous and ask her friends to come along. When one of the girls laughed at her, saying that she was "weird" for wanting to go to "that" movie, and everyone else, including her best friend Rachel, joined in with the taunt, something snapped inside Abigail. She finally realized that her friends were not her friends. Abigail told Miriam about what had happened, and relayed the hurt she felt about the girls taunting her and that Rachel hadn't stood up for her. Miriam, the compromising peacemaker, responded by suggesting that Abigail see the situation from Rachel's perspective. That perhaps Rachel didn't want to lose face in front of their friends, or was trying to be a peacemaker and defuse the situation.

During their next session, Abigail said to her mother, "What you said really hurt me. You completely ignored my feelings. You told me I should forget how Rachel's lack of support felt, and worry more about how my suggestion that we go and see the movie had upset everyone. I don't understand why you took her side. You're my mom. You're supposed to be on my side."

After an awkward silence, she said to Miriam, "When did you stop being honest? When did you start becoming so afraid of upsetting people?"

Miriam looked visibly shocked by Abigail's accusation. And after a moment in which I could tell Miriam was reflecting on Abigail's words, she said, "You're right, honey, I'm not honest with my friends. Our therapy has really shown me this, and it's a hard thing to know about myself. I don't even think I'm always totally honest with your dad. I'm far too worried about upsetting people that I forget myself. I know I have to work on this."

Pontus had been listening, watching the exchange, and spoke up. "Yeah, I feel hurt when you don't tell me what you're really thinking," he said to Miriam. "Don't you think I know when something's bothering you? When you brush me off when I ask you what's wrong, you make me feel as if I don't matter to you."

After a tearful silence, Miriam said, "You're both right. Mom used to say that relationships require compromise. I guess what she meant was that as a woman, I should do all the compromising. Mom spent her life trying to make people happy. It made her happy when she made someone happy. But I didn't realize until now how much Mom defined her own happiness through other people's happiness. When I was young, I used to hate it when she would make me see an argument I was having with my friends from my friend's perspective. And now I'm doing the same to you. This has to stop. I don't want to repeat that with you."

Creating Generational Change

A few sessions later, Abigail came to her session looking radiant. She had just defriended her friends off Facebook because the previous Saturday evening, her friends had bullied her on Facebook by making up stories about her because she hadn't gone with them to the movies. Abigail didn't go because she was tired, but also because she didn't like the boys her friends were going with. She wanted to stay at home and chill out and watch a movie on Netflix. She knew her friends wouldn't like that she hadn't joined them, but she didn't care. She no longer wanted to compromise herself for their comfort.

Talking about what happened, she said, "I hadn't realized how bored I was with my friends. All they talk about is boys and makeup. I'm sick of it. And they behaved really badly last weekend, so I'm done with them. I feel sad that Rachel decided to side with them, but I can't help that. Maybe Rachel wasn't such a good friend after all."

Using the exercises below and the maxims you'll read about in the next chapter (Chapter 8), Miriam and Abigail worked on communicating what they thought, felt, and needed. I gave them the homework exercise that taught them how to *understand what it is like to be in each other's shoes.* This exercise, which I use with many of my clients, is based on Solution 1 of the *Mother-Daughter Coaching Model* (outlined in Chapter 4). That solution explains that mothers and daughters are people first, with ideas, experiences, and needs of their own, and it teaches mothers and daughters to listen to, and accept, each other's unfiltered truth, even if one's truth varies widely or clashes with the other's.

I find that when mothers and daughters share their unfiltered, emotional truth about the sacrifices they have had to make, the needs that weren't met, and how life situations and role stereotypes limited their choices, blame and guilt evaporate. When Miriam told Abigail how hard it was for her, and her grandmother, to be a female doctor in a male-dominated profession, Abigail's attitude toward her mother softened. She gained a greater appreciation for how her mother had to create a certain persona, just to survive in her male-dominated profession. And with new eyes, Abigail saw how Miriam had tried her best as a mother, even though at times she hadn't provided the emotional caring Abigail needed. Miriam had tried to meet everyone's needs at work and at home, and what Miriam needed, and sometimes what Abigail needed, had gotten lost in the crush.

During their last sessions, Miriam and Abigail discussed how women lose themselves in their relationships too easily, and how they were going to create a new normal where they would be free to be themselves and define their own lives. This was going to be an exciting journey of discovery for them, which would inevitably cause them to feel some heartache, as Abigail had already discovered. Miriam too had learned that some of her colleagues didn't like her newfound honesty. Miriam and Abigail were pioneers, pushing themselves, and the women around them, into the next stage of women's evolution, where mothers and daughters are people first. They wanted to pass on all they had learned through their couple's therapy by creating a *Women's Power Circle* at Abigail's school for mothers and daughters. (You'll learn about these Power Circles in Chapter 9.) They wanted to empower other mothers and daughters to join them in shattering the age-old expectations of sacrifice, self-denial, and self-silencing, and create a new balance for women where women listen, speak, lead, and follow, and care for, and are cared for, in equal measures.

Exercise: Advocating For What You Need

The process of learning how to speak what you need emotionally is much like the practice of mindfulness. The instructions are simple, but the practice is hard. The instructions for the practice of mindfulness is to simply return to your breath, and focus on how your breath feels in your body when you inevitably go off on some thought tangent in your mind. Anyone who has tried to practice mindfulness knows how difficult this is. Our minds wander with the slightest provocation. But if we dedicate ourselves to this practice, we reap the numerous wellbeing benefits it promises.

Learning how to identify what you are feeling and emotionally need, and being comfortable voicing it, follows much the same pattern. The instructions are simply to ask, "What am I feeling and what do I need?" And if you don't know the answer to these questions, don't beat yourself up. Similar to the practice of mindfulness, it takes dedicated practice to strengthen this emotional muscle. The conversation that inquires after and honors what you feel and emotionally need is like a muscle that goes slack with lack of use. The more you ask this question, the stronger the muscle will become, and the easier the answers come, and the more you reap the emotional benefits of knowing yourself.

Following is a list of questions that build on from the chapter and the exercises on claiming your needs in *The Silent Female Scream*,[3] that help women identify when they are silencing themselves or being silenced. I suggest that you journal your answers every day. The more you ask these questions, the easier the answers will come, and eventually, they will be second nature.

1. What am I feeling today?
2. What do I need emotionally?
3. Did I voice how I felt today? If so, how did it feel? If not, why not? Did it feel safe or unsafe? Was I afraid that I wouldn't be heard, or did I doubt that I had the right to speak?
4. Did I voice what I emotionally needed today? If so, how did it feel? If not, why not? Did it feel safe or unsafe? Was I afraid that I wouldn't be heard, or did I doubt that I had the right to be emotionally honest?
5. What do I need to do tomorrow so that I voice my truth?
6. What do I need to do when someone doesn't inquire after what I'm thinking or feeling, or when they don't listen to me?

Exercise: Write Your Own Bill of Emotional Rights

The following exercise empowers women to live by their personal Bill of Emotional Rights. We all need to have our own emotional code by which we live, and I give this exercise to my clients, as well as to the women who join my *Women's Power Circles* (see Chapter 9). This exercise is best done in pairs, or in a supportive circle of women, because it is through the discussion of each other's Bill of Emotional Rights that we learn how to raise our beliefs in what we are entitled to.

Writing your Bill of Emotional Rights is a good exercise to do after you finish mapping your mother-daughter history (See instructions in Chapter 6). Go back to the list you made in your *Mother-Daughter History Map* of the sexist and emotionally disempowering themes and patterns in your generational family that you recorded in Step 8, where you worked on creating a roadmap for change. Use this list to write a list of positive behaviors and expectations you will now live by.

Write each statement as an "I" statement, a declaration that positively states the behavior you now want to engage in. For example: "I will check in with how I'm feeling and what is right for me whenever someone asks me to do something."

I gave Miriam and Abigail this exercise after we mapped Miriam's mother-daughter history. Her roadmap for change listed the following harmful generational themes or patterns.

1. Women do not voice their own needs.
2. Women take too much responsibility for other people's needs and too little for their own.
3. Women are invisible as people in their own right.
4. Women are self-denying and overaccommodating.

Miriam and Abigail took these four themes and turned them into the following Bill of Emotional Rights.

1. Every day I will check in with how I'm feeling and what I need emotionally.
2. Every morning I will review whether I was emotionally honest the day before. And if I find that I wasn't honest when I wanted to be, I will explore what was going on in that moment, and in the moments before it, that resulted in me staying silent.
3. Before I do something for someone, I will check whether it feels like a "hallelujah yes," a "not sure," or a resounding "no." And I will only follow up and agree to do something if it feels like a hallelujah yes.
4. I will not agree to do anything that feels too much, or too much of a personal compromise.
5. Before I commit to a friendship, I will check if they are willing and able to listen to, and respect, my feelings and emotional needs.
6. I will walk away from any relationship that is not reciprocated.

Miriam and Abigail put a copy of their Bill of Emotional Rights up on their refrigerator, so they could remind themselves, and each other, of the standard they now live by. After about six months of daily reminders, they no longer needed to have it on their refrigerator because their Bill of Emotional Rights had become second nature to them.

In the next chapter, I outline six maxims I used in my work with Miriam and Abigail, and with my other clients, that raise women's emotional entitlement to not do all the emotional work in their relationships.

CHAPTER 8

CHANGING GENERATIONAL PATTERNS OF SEXISM

We live in a world that is reluctant to make room for women.

IN 2013, I accompanied my husband to Istanbul where he attended a conference for small and medium-sized business owners. At the end of the conference I was invited to join him, along with the other conference delegates and their wives, on a cruise down the Bosphorus Strait. It was a glorious day. The scenery was spectacular and the villas sparkled in the sunlight. But it wasn't the scenery that stole my attention. I became fixated on observing how the men had spread themselves out throughout the entire deck of the boat. I kept watching a group of men who sat in classic "manspreading" style along the stern, which was the best place to see the views, while their wives and girlfriends sat below deck, or in tightly squeezed groups along the sides of the boat. On the way back, I was shocked to see how again the men commanded all the best seats while their wives and girlfriends sat unobtrusively in whatever spaces that were left over.

As I reflected on why the men felt so entitled to inhabit whatever space they desired (and why there were so few female business owners on the cruise), I wondered if this scene would have looked any different had the conference been in France, Germany, England, or America, and the cruise down the Rhine, Thames, or Mississippi. Would there have been more women delegates? Would the male delegates still have usurped the best seats on the boat? Would the men have been as oblivious about their wives' right to enjoy the cruise in comfort, as the men were on this cruise? And would the wives have tolerated being relegated to inferior viewing places?

Most conference delegates on this cruise were men from Turkey, India, Pakistan, and African countries, and I imagine that had the conference been in another country, there would have been more female business owners and the space on the boat would have been more equally divided between the men and women. Regardless of these differences, the women on the cruise represented for me how women everywhere struggle to claim enough space for themselves. They reminded me of how I instinctively made way for men when I was walking down the street, and how some men expected me to move over for them. How when I was lane swimming at my local swimming pool, I had to watch out for certain male swimmers because they would kick me if I didn't move over for them. How on public transport, I saw men looking more comfortable with taking up space than women. In conversations, I heard men speak more often than women. I saw women hesitating before they spoke, and apologizing before they had even said anything. I saw women masking their voice as they held their hands in front of their mouths. And I heard women grieving about how little time, consideration, and focus they were receiving from their husbands.

Even though my mother and grandmother were Dutch, I can imagine they would have behaved just like the women on the cruise. My grandmother would have encouraged her husband to take the best seat on the boat, while she contented herself with an inferior one. She would have fussed over him, bringing him food and drink, and had her son joined her, she would have treated him with the same servitude. My Dutch grandfather would also have behaved like the men on the cruise. He wouldn't have given his wife's needs a moment's thought or asked whether she was enjoying herself. All my grandfather cared about was his own enjoyment. To him, if he was having fun so was his wife, because in his mind, his enjoyment was also hers.

I don't know if any of the women on the cruise silently protested to themselves about their unfair treatment, but I know that my mother would have protested had she been on the cruise as a girl. My mother would have been expected to follow her mother's lead and allow her father and brother to take the best seats. But judging from the stories my grandmother has told me about my mother when she was a girl, I think my mother would have rebelled. I can imagine my mother as a young woman, rushing to the back of the boat and claiming the best spot for herself, because back then she had a strong sense of fairness. And I can also imagine the outrage she would have felt when her parents made her forfeit her seat to her father and brother and then criticize her for being a greedy, disobedient girl.

It feels sad reminiscing about how my mother was taught to not prioritize herself, and to silence her built-in hatred of unfairness and inequality when she was a girl. I can see how this lesson wounded her. How it turned her into a bitter, jealous person who hated seeing anyone, especially me as her daughter, get whatever she wasn't allowed to have as a child, and whatever she didn't allow herself to do as an adult. I know that had I been on the cruise as a girl, I too would have rushed to claim the best seat, and my mother would have behaved just like my grandmother. She would have instructed me to give up my seat to my father and brother, and she would have chastised me for being a greedy girl, just as her mother would have.

This theme of squashing women's built-in resistance against unfair and unequal treatment is a very old generational pattern in my family. It forms the metaphorical shoes mothers and daughters wear and the beliefs and expectations mothers pass on to daughters. And I believe that this generational pattern led my great-grandmother to become a little crazy, my grandmother to become stoic, and my mother angry and controlling. Sadly, my mother wore those behavior traits like a protective armor I was never able to pierce.

My great-grandmother was a missionary's wife in Indonesia, and was expected to sacrifice her life for her husband's calling. This meant saying goodbye to each of her children when they turned six years old, because they were sent back to Holland for their education. There is a story in my family of how my great-grandmother became haunted by the eyes of one of her son's teddy bears. She felt that the teddy bear's eyes were staring back at her in an accusing way, from the ashes of a bonfire they had of the boy's belongings after he was put on a ship destined for Holland. I can only imagine the unvoiced pain my great-grandmother must have felt each time she said goodbye to her child, and how she must have struggled to bond with her babies, knowing that she would only mother them for six short years.

My grandmother too was expected to be of service to her husband. This meant shutting her eyes to his bullying behavior, and to his infidelity and incest. From the stories I've heard, and from my experience of having known my grandfather during his later years, I know that my grandmother's marriage wasn't a happy one. My grandfather was quite similar to my great-grandfather. Both men were controlling, opinionated, and highly patriarchal in their unquestioned entitlement to do whatever they pleased without having to consider their wives' needs or wishes. My grandmother must have married my grandfather because he felt strangely familiar to her, even though his behavior wasn't kind or caring. And getting a divorce was unthinkable in her day. In her family, divorce was a mark of the wife's failure to keep her marriage together, and thus her shaming the family. My grandmother and her sisters learned to buckle under these beliefs and "make the best of it," as my grandmother used to say.

The story of my grandmother's marriage reflects the emotional neglect she suffered from throughout her entire life. Having spent her life surrounded by controlling, patriarchal men and silent, submissive women who dutifully complied with their father's and husband's wishes, and who swallowed their rage about their unvoiced feelings and needs, my grandmother never learned to expect anything different.

I don't think my grandmother was ever exposed to a woman who voiced her feelings and needs in an upfront and honest way, and if she had, I'm sure she wouldn't have liked her. In my grandmother's family environment, it would have been nearly impossible for her to copy this emotionally empowered woman's behavior, because she would have suffered from the same consequences as Sandeep did in Chapter 3. My grandmother would have been expelled from her family.

This is the legacy, or metaphorical shoes, my mother inherited from her mother, and sadly, her generation didn't help her find a better-fitting pair. The post–Second World War era my mother came of age in guilt-tripped her into believing that having a paid job alongside being a mother and wife was wrong. Women during that time were pressured to give up their jobs to returning servicemen, and return to their "God-given" role as all-giving, financially dependent mothers and wives, and my mother took on this role entirely, though it was a bad fit for her. Too much childhood neglect from her emotionally unavailable mother, and two years in a Japanese concentration camp in Indonesia during the war when she was only ten years old, left her emotionally unable to recognize the harmful beliefs she had internalized and choose a different path for herself.

This generational emotional reality created enmeshed mother-daughter relationships in my family. My mother and grandmother spent their lives emotionally glued to their unhappy and emotionally mute mothers, and I was expected to do the same. But from a young age I knew that my survival, and my children's survival, hinged on me changing the harmful generational patterns in my family and finding a new way of relating to myself and my mother. I didn't want my daughter's built-in resistance to unfair and unequal treatment to be squashed. I didn't want to limit her choices and freedom. I didn't want to emotionally glue her to me, hence making her responsible for my unmet needs and happiness. And I wanted my daughter and I, and women everywhere, to recognize emotional silencing and gender inequality for what they are, and together create a world where women are a priority, and where women know how to prioritize themselves.

Looking back, I can see how I started my journey in changing my harmful inherited patterns from a place of extreme naivety. Like all of us,

I didn't know what I didn't know, and not knowing made me vulnerable to recreating my inherited dysfunction and emotional disempowerment in my marriage and friendships. Like Miriam and Abigail (in Chapter 7), people liked me because I was, and am, a good listener. But I needed to wake myself up to the extreme level of invisibility I had become accustomed to, and learn to be comfortable with being heard, seen, and nurtured. And like Sandeep (in Chapter 3), I had to come to terms with my mother's anger, and being expelled from my family, because I was breaking my family's rules of what it means to be female.

Throughout my own journey of awakening and through my work with women, I've developed the following six maxims that challenge the invisibility women have inherited from previous generations. Like most women, I had to learn that relationships are like bridges, as maxim number one teaches, that require *both* people to make equal effort in building a reciprocal relationship. I had to recognize the many ways sexism and patriarchy like to guilt-trip women into keeping quiet. How sexism likes to point the finger of blame away from the sexist ways it treats women back to the victim, by making her feel guilty. We see this reflection in action when a rape victim is asked what she was wearing, or a battered wife is asked what she did to make her husband angry, or an abused daughter is asked what she did to make her mother angry with her. And I needed to learn that voicing my opinions and needs wasn't an aggressive stance, as maxim six teaches, but a life-affirming one that gives me the right to walk away from anyone who doesn't know how to listen.

The following six maxims create a firewall around the Culture of Female Service by raising women's entitlement to need, be heard, set boundaries, and have reciprocal relationships. They teach women how to say no without feeling guilty, to ask questions without feeling ashamed, to not take on another person's anger when it isn't theirs to own, and to not be tricked into believing the age-old sexism that punishes women when they don't comply with their own silencing.

Relationships Are Like a Bridge

This maxim challenges the age-old patriarchal belief that makes women responsible for doing all the emotional work in relationships, by comparing relationships to building a bridge. A bridge is built from each side until it meets in the middle at the keystone, which holds the bridge up. You cannot build a bridge by building it up from one side, and then carrying on through the keystone, and then building it down the other side. That is structurally impossible. Relationships are no different. A woman cannot build a relationship in which she is heard and supported by trying to do all the listening and caring. That is an emotional impossibility. She needs the other person to perform their equal share of being emotionally available, so that together they can build a relationship that recognizes both of their voices and both of their needs.

This maxim applies to all relationships. It applies to women's love relationships, girlfriend relationships, work relationships, and mother-and-adult-daughter relationships. It teaches women, through the following questions, how to change patterns of emotional neglect by becoming aware of how they feel about their relationships, and to stop feeling responsible for what the other person brings or doesn't bring to the relationship.

1. How do I feel about my relationships? Do I feel heard, or do I have to fight to be heard?
2. Am I feeling exhausted and all given-out?
3. Do I keep quiet about things that are important to me because I don't feel confident about speaking up, or am I in relationships with people who aren't interested in listening to my point of view?
4. Do I feel loved for being me, or am I trying to be loved by giving extra love and support?

Relationships Are a Two-Way Street

This maxim continues to teach women that a good relationship is a reciprocal one, where both people listen and feel heard, and give and receive.

There are many ways to describe this maxim. Some clients respond to a more financial-themed idiom like, "Am I getting the emotional return I need from my investment in this relationship?" Others prefer a more sensory one like, "Am I feeding from crumbs of attention and pretending the crumb is a cake?" And others like, "Am I forgetting to, or feeling afraid to, advocate for what I need in my relationships?"

The questions below help women change patterns of emotional silence and emotional neglect, and they stop women from repeatedly giving from a place of empty and misreading crumbs of attention.

1. Is the listening, caring, and support I provide being reciprocated, or do my requests to be heard fall on deaf ears? Do I have to beg or scream to be heard?
2. If I have to beg or scream to be heard, what am I doing with my hurt feelings about not being heard? Do I ignore my hurt feelings and refocus my attention on being more supportive, with the hope that one day my efforts will be reciprocated? Or do I explain away the person's neglectful behavior by making excuses for them about why they aren't able to be emotionally available?
3. Do I have a tendency to feed from crumbs of attention and pretend that the crumb is bigger than it is?
4. How do I replenish the emotional well from which I give? Who provides me with love and a listening ear?

Three-Second Rule

This maxim addresses the oceans of guilt mothers feel that isn't theirs. The following questions challenge the misogyny of mother-blaming by reminding women that there are two different types of guilt. The first type is real guilt. This guilt or shame is felt when we deliberately or inadvertently hurt someone. This guilt is healthy, because without it, we're in danger of being a sociopath. The second type is toxic guilt. Women feel this guilt or shame when they go against a code of behavior that patriarchy has set out for them.

Toxic guilt is felt when a woman feels bad for not doing enough, even though she isn't getting what she needs in return. Another example is when a woman feels bad for speaking up, even though her thoughts haven't been inquired after or welcomed. Or when she feels selfish for doing what is best for her, and she's feeling shame or guilt for going against the Culture of Female Service code, which expects her to sacrifice her needs for the good of others.

Feeling selfish is a classic example of toxic guilt. I believe that the word "selfish" has lost all its original meaning, in terms of someone behaving in a truly self-centered, disrespectful way that neglects others people's rights and needs. The irony is that this definition describes how patriarchy treats women. Patriarchal thinking is selfish, and is neglectful of what women need. And it uses the guilt-tripping, shame-inducing accusation of being selfish to deflect women's (and men's) attention away from the inherent selfishness in patriarchal thinking, and co-opting women into complying with their own neglect.

Here is how the *three-second rule* works.

1. Can I come up with a real crime that I've committed in three seconds or less? If I can't, then the guilt I'm feeling is toxic and not for me to own.
2. What toxic guilt am I feeling? What sexist or patriarchal rule or belief have I broken?
3. Now that I recognize the sexist rule or belief I've broken, I must congratulate myself for having spoken up, for not tolerating being dismissed, and for demanding that I am heard and respected, and celebrate with my plain-speaking female relatives and girlfriends.

Guilt by Proxy

This maxim follows the *three-second rule* by teaching women to turn the finger of blame away from themselves to the person or society that perpetrated the crime. Guilt by proxy exposes the guilt and shame society bears for the way it doesn't protect and respect women's rights and needs. It reveals how a conspiracy of silence about the way a person or society has mistreated a woman leaves the victimized woman silenced and forgotten, and shouldering the blame for how she was abused or mistreated. It reveals how within this conspiracy of silence, where a woman's anger isn't heard or acknowledged, toxic guilt flourishes. Silence points the finger of blame at the victim rather than at the perpetrator, which adds another layer of victimization on the victim. When women are empowered to not take responsibility for other people's crimes, toxic blame and guilt evaporate. Women stop feeling like a victim, and the real perpetrator is made to account for their crime whether they acknowledge it or not.

An example of this silencing is happening right now in American universities. American universities have been shockingly slow in taking responsibility for the culture of rape that is epidemic on their campuses, as described in the book and movie *The Hunting Ground*.[1] Female victims are being pressured to keep silent and question their own behavior, and accept that universities feel more responsible for protecting their own brand than providing a safe environment for their female students. In this example, guilt by proxy and the three-second rule teaches female college students to not feel responsible for being raped or assaulted—to point the finger of blame away from themselves and back toward the perpetrator, and the university, for having created an organizational culture where the rape and assault of female students is tolerated.

Here is how *guilt by proxy* works.

1. Identify a crime that has been committed against you, or a moment when someone hurt your feelings, and think about who committed the crime or hurt your feelings.
2. In three seconds, try to come up with a solid reason why you deserve to be hurt or mistreated.
3. When you cannot come up with a solid reason—which you won't, because it doesn't include being a selfish, ungrateful person, or that you were out alone, drunk, or wearing a short skirt—create a ritual that passes back the responsibility for the violation or the hurt to the person who perpetrated it. Be creative! Make the ritual meaningful, so that it

has the power to absolve you from feeling guilt that isn't yours to own. I like to write the person's name and their crime on a piece of paper and then burn it, so it disappears back into the atmosphere.

4. Now create a mantra that is meaningful to you, one you can invoke whenever you feel guilt by proxy. The mantras I have used in the past are: "my feelings matter"; "I am enough"; and, "other people's choices and behaviors having nothing to do with me."

Three Strikes and You're Out

This maxim was inspired by one of Maya Angelou's wisdoms, from an interview I watched on the *Oprah Winfrey Show*: "When someone shows you who they are, believe them." It gives women permission to walk away when someone is being dismissive of their feelings and needs, or downright emotionally abusive. Too many women are carrying a deep, weeping wound on their souls because the love and care they have given hasn't been reciprocated. This kind of wound can smart with fearful thoughts that, maybe, she is not worth loving.

The following questions empower women to not keep dismissing or ignoring hurtful or abusive behavior, and to walk away from an abusive relationship or an emotionally neglecting relationship that is robbing them of their love and energy.

1. Take notice of how someone behaves toward you and how his or her behavior feels.
2. If, after three times, they show through their words or behavior, or their lack of words and behavior, that they don't know how to behave in a respectful, caring, mutually supportive way, walk away. If the person is emotionally or physically abusive, they only get *one* strike before they are out and you walk away. They don't deserve a second chance!
3. Walk away believing that this isn't your fault. Believe that this person isn't relationship material. That they don't know how to be emotionally present in a relationship, and that your soul and your emotional wellbeing needs and deserves better than they can provide.

4. If you can't walk away entirely because it's a family member who is being neglectful, limit your involvement to match, as closely as you can, the level of emotional availability they are giving. This is an important step to remember, because it protects you from becoming emotionally exhausted and feeling robbed or used.

Assertive Is Not the Same as Aggressive

This maxim corrects the misconception that when a woman is being assertive, she is only one step away from being aggressive, which isn't true. Aggressive behavior stems from an entirely different emotional state than assertive behavior does. Assertive behavior comes from an emotionally strong place. When a woman is being assertive, she is speaking from a place that knows she has a right to be heard and she doesn't need anyone to validate this. Aggressive behavior, by contrast, comes from an emotionally disempowered place. When a woman is being aggressive she is behaving from a fearful place that is worried she won't be heard. And if we knew something about her life, her worry about not being heard is likely to stem from real experiences where her voice and needs were silenced or dismissed. She would have learned, through these hurtful experiences, and from her generational family, that the only way to get noticed is through being aggressive.

Another aspect of this maxim is that it shatters the perception that aggressive behavior is always loud, forceful, and angry. This is not the case. The more quiet behaviors of being a martyr, or an emotional manipulator, are also aggressive, emotionally bullying behaviors, which stem from the same fear that a person's needs and voice won't be heard.

The following questions help increase your assertive behavior.

1. What are you keeping quiet about? What are you afraid to say?
2. Who told you not to talk about it or ask for it?
3. What are you afraid will happen if you speak up or ask for what you need? How will people react? Who do you think will be angry with you?

4. Imagine that you have spoken up, and the person you thought would be angry, is. Go to the *three-second rule* and check to see if you've committed a real crime. Why is the person acting as if you've committed a crime for advocating for your right to have your thoughts, feelings, and needs heard and honored? What does their anger say about their ability to listen to you and see you as your own person who they can't and should not control? And if this was happening to your daughter or friend, would you want them to keep quiet, or would you encourage them to speak up? Do your voice and needs matter as much as your daughter's or friend's?

In the next chapter, I tell the story of four women who have gathered in a *Women's Power Circle* I am facilitating. As these women talk about how they silence themselves, how they comply with limiting gender roles and the Culture of Female Service, and how they tolerate emotional neglect in their relationships, they are emboldened to speak and be heard, and take back their right to make their own decisions about their lives.

CHAPTER 9

STRENGTHENING ALL FEMALE RELATIONSHIPS

When women and girls are heard and emotionally supported, they are more able to listen to and mutually support each other.

I EXPERIENCED A POWERFUL moment of women being emotionally honest while I was teaching a class on sexism and gender roles at Nottingham Trent University in England. A female student said, "It isn't the men we have to watch out for, it's other women." No sooner had she said this, the entire class of female undergraduate students roared in agreement. It was painful to hear how these young women had already learned to not trust each other. That they had experienced, on too many occasions, how women hold each other to the same sexist standards they have co-opted from society. Yet I was also pleased that the women felt safe enough in the class to voice this truth, especially since women rarely talk about women's sexist behavior toward each other.

As the analysis throughout this book shows, talking about how women act out the sexism they have internalized isn't victim blaming, as many feminists fear. Nor does it distract from making men accountable for their sexist behavior. Rather, the opposite. It exposes how sexism and gender inequality sets not just mothers and daughters up for conflict, but all female relationships. It reveals how all woman-to-woman conflict, whether between a mother and daughter, girlfriends, work colleagues, or in women's groups or circles, is a window into the sexism that women have internalized from their families and sociocultural environment.

It makes sense that women and girls will treat each other in the same way they themselves are treated. As pictured in the diagram below, when women connect as friends or colleagues, or in groups, they bring to the relationship, or group, their individual mother-daughter history and the beliefs and gender stereotypes they inherited from their mother, multigenerational family, and sociocultural environment. Similar to mothers and daughters, when women haven't learned how to speak what they feel, think, and need, they don't know how to listen to or speak this language with their girlfriends, work colleagues, or women's groups. And similar to mothers and daughters, women will silence each other in the same way they have learned to silence themselves.

SOLVING THE FEMALE RELATIONSHIP PUZZLE

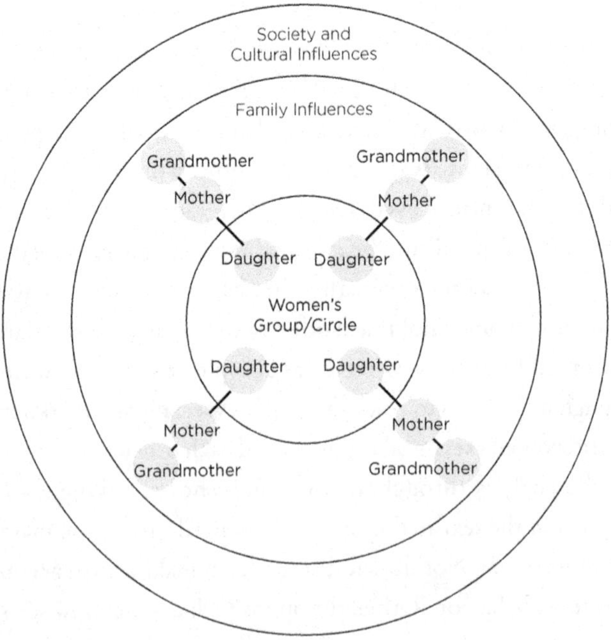

We all know the subtle, guilt-tripping ways women silence each other. The "no response" silencing that makes a woman worry that she hasn't been heard, or worse, that she has said or done something wrong. The "what about me?" silencing, where a woman talks endlessly about herself without listening to others, because she is starving-hungry to be heard. The "surely you don't mean that," or "you're overreacting" silencing that questions a woman's emotional truth and makes her feel wrong for feeling the way she does. The "why don't you think about what the other person is feeling?" as Miriam (in Chapter 7) asked her daughter Abigail to do when Abigail's friend didn't stand up for her, only serves to reinforce the stereotype that a likeable woman is self-silencing, and she shouldn't make other women accountable for the hurt they've caused. The "don't you worry about the other person?" silencing also questions a woman's right to say no, to set boundaries, and to own her feelings. And, finally, women silence their own and each other's unique perspectives and emotional reality, because they've learned to see themselves through an internalized male lens and suppress their voices underneath what men think and need.

Here, I'll continue Sandeep's story (from Chapter 3) as she joins a *Women's Power Circle* I facilitated and learns how to have emotionally honest and mutually supportive relationships with the other women in her circle. *Women's Power Circles* are small groups of women or girls that meet weekly for six weeks. I developed *Women's Power Circles* back in 2008 for three reasons. First, I wanted to create a space where women supported each other as they explored their mother-daughter history, strengthened their entitlement to speak, be heard, and claim their emotional needs, and changed harmful sexist beliefs and cultural patterns. Second, I wanted to create a space where women saw for themselves their shared generational experiences with emotional silence and emotional neglect. And third, I wanted to create a space where, unlike my Springboard experience in Chapter 3, women didn't silence themselves, or each other.

As the *Mother-Daughter Coaching Model* explains, female relationships where women are heard, emotionally supported, and free to be themselves, aren't created as if by magic. They require an agreement that women are people first, and that underneath the arguments and conflict lies the all-important generational theme of how women need to feel entitled to, and encouraged to, speak what they need and prioritize their physical and emotional wellbeing. I believe that when we understand that women the world over have inherited their mother's experience of emotional silencing and emotional neglect, women's circles become spaces where women can bond over their shared history. When this is understood, women's circles become spaces where women really listen to themselves, and each other, where they give each other permission to be self-nurturing, where they support each other's goals and dreams, and where women become a powerful force for change.

Women's Power Circle Story

This *Women's Power Circle* story is from the second week of the six-week experience, where the topic of conversation was how to claim what you need. Sandeep (from Chapter 3), Samantha, Britney, and Danielle met in my office on Wednesday evenings. They had each joined the circle because they needed to raise their entitlement to speak and be heard, and they needed to be supported as they struggled with their particular problems and issues.

Sandeep joined the circle because she needed to surround herself with a supportive group of women who could help her as she navigated the difficult transition to prioritizing her life and career from her caretaking role. Samantha, a fifty-five-year-old stay-at-home mother and wife, joined the circle because her doctor had recommended it. He was hoping that a *Women's Power Circle* experience would help her find out why she was suffering from headaches and joint pains that had no medical diagnosis. As Samantha entered the room for the first circle meeting, I could see her pain etched on her face. Britney, a thirty-year-old professional, arrived dressed in her business suit, having come straight from work. Britney had joined the circle because she needed to leave her abusive boyfriend. Her boyfriend was paranoid about women in his past relationships cheating on him, and he constantly questioned Britney about where she was going and who she was seeing. And Danielle, a thirty-three-year-old mother of two young children who had recently left her husband, joined the circle because she needed support while she filed for divorce.

The week before, the women had introduced themselves to each other and mapped their mother-daughter histories. In brief, Sandeep had shared some details of how demanding and guilt-tripping her mother was, and her struggle with juggling her family's demands and her studies. She had talked about the severe emotional neglect from which the women in her multigenerational family had suffered. Samantha shared that she was at a point in her life where she was tired of taking care of people, and wanted to learn how to say no without feeling guilty. Through her mother-daughter history, she discovered how deeply the "selfless caring" role ran in her multigenerational family, and that right from college she had stepped into her mother's and grandmother's shoes. Britney had talked about being guilt-tripped by her verbally abusive boyfriend and her discovery that generation after generation, the women in her family fell in love with abusive men. And finally, Danielle shared her feelings of guilt about the dearth of time her children spent with their father, even though she knew she had no power over her husband's relationship with his kids. And in her *Mother-Daughter History Map*, she had found an answer she was looking for that explained why her mother and mother-in-law weren't being supportive of her decision to leave her husband.

Circle Meeting Begins

The women arrived for their meeting excited about gathering with their new friends. I noticed, though, that Danielle was looking upset about something. As I opened the circle by lighting a candle, I said the following words.

"In this circle we are all equal and equally important. We are here to learn about how to speak our minds rather than keep silent. We are here to learn how to advocate for ourselves, rather than follow what others expect from us. We are here to learn that speaking our truth and acting in our best interest is not inconsistent with being cooperative and collaborative. We are here to understand how the silencing of women's needs has taught women to be emotionally manipulative. In this circle, we will learn how to use our power in direct ways. We will speak our truth, we will look at ourselves and each other with nonjudgmental eyes, and we will support each other as we connect the dots between our choices and how we behave and how our family, and society, treats women."

After a short pause I concluded the opening with, "A woman who is surrounded by a circle of permission-giving women who encourage her to do what is best and right for her has found a soft place in which to feel powerful."

Recalling Danielle's earlier demeanor, I invited her to start the conversation by asking her how she was feeling.

"I'm really angry," she said with undisguised ire in her voice. "My husband, sorry, my soon-to-be ex-husband called me about an hour ago to tell me he couldn't have the kids tonight. Our agreement was that he has the kids on Wednesday evenings, and suddenly he calls me at six, to tell me he has to go to a presentation from a visiting professor. Like he didn't know that earlier," she added with increasing volume. "And of course he couldn't possibly not attend."

"How bloody typical of him," she continued. "This is how he is. He has no regard for what I need, or that his kids are looking forward to spending time with him. His work is all he sees, and he gets angry if we don't understand this. He makes us fit in with him. His dad was the same. His mom fit her entire life around his father. Well I'll be damned if I'm going to do that. I don't want to repeat my mother-in-law's life, and I don't want my daughter and son to grow up thinking the world revolves around men."

As she spat out her words, she revealed the pain she felt about having invested years of her life in loving and supporting a man who didn't reciprocate her love and support. I knew from last week's meeting that Danielle's mother and mother-in-law weren't supportive of her decision to leave her husband. In her family and her in-law family, the women were emotionally starved. They had learned to feed from the occasional crumb of attention from their husbands. And Danielle's newly raised expectations, that her husband should listen to her and support her as a person in her own right, was an uncomfortable mirror for either family to look at. They didn't want to see their emotionally neglected lives staring back at them through Danielle's decision to leave her husband, so they had teamed up, with the hope that their united front would force Danielle to reverse her decision and return to her husband.

Danielle shifted in her chair, looked around our circle, and said, "I'm amazed by how supported I felt last week. I've never had my thoughts and feelings affirmed like this before. Thank you for listening and really understanding. Since last week, something fundamental has changed in my mind. I now know, without a shadow of doubt, that the way my husband neglects me, and ignores me, is wrong. I can no longer go back to tolerating his neglectful behavior, and giving great gobs of effort in the hope he'll hear me."

Everyone laughed at her description of "great gobs of effort," and her expression lightened for a moment. "And," she continued with another look around, "you helped me see that my family's, and my in-laws' accusations that I'm being selfish, self-centered, and a dishonorable wife is complete rubbish. I now see how upside down their idea of an honorable wife is, how it denies any responsibility for my rights and life."

"I love how you said that, 'great gobs of effort,'" said Samantha. "That's going to stick in my mind next time I'm giving *great gobs of effort* in the hope that my husband and mother will notice me."

"Me too," Sandeep said.

The chuckles faded quickly, though, and Danielle continued. "Talking to all of you has made something shift for me. Before, when my husband let me down I'd end up in a tailspin. His accusations that I'm demanding, or not supportive of how hard he works for his family . . . that used to mess up my mind and make me feel unsure about whether I had a right to ask him to take care of the children. But tonight? I've taken a step back from his guilt-tripping. Tonight, I don't believe him when he says he works hard for the family. He's obsessed with his career. He's ambitious. That's what drives him, not his family."

"Yeah," everyone said in unison, because most of them had dealt with similar accusations and situations.

"I'm so glad to hear you say that," said Samantha. "Your husband sounds selfish, and what you said opened my eyes to how my husband behaves. He says the same things about how hard he works for all of us, and he does work hard, but it isn't just for the family. He works hard because he's ambitious. Like you, I'm wondering if it's wrong that I've been expected to sacrifice my life and dreams on the altar of his ambition."

"You're right, it is wrong, Samantha," Danielle said. "No wife should sacrifice her needs for her husband's ambition."

"It is wonderful to hear how solid you sound tonight," I said to Danielle. "You're decontaminating yourself of your husband's voice, and your family and in-law family's voices. You're seeing clearly how your husband, family, and in-law family want you to step back in line with their belief in the Culture of Female Service, and ignore how invisible it makes you feel. There's another dynamic too. This one's happening between you and your mother and mother-in-law. They want you to step back in line and walk a repeat of their lives, so they don't have to look through your choices at what they have had to do without."

Turning to Sandeep I said, "I guess you know what it's like to walk in Danielle's shoes?"

Sandeep nodded. "Sure do. Last week I came home determined to give my studies the time they deserve. Like you, Danielle, a gap has formed between what I want, and what my parents want me to want. I think the best way to describe it is that they no longer feel right up against my face." Sandeep put her hands up against her face as she said this.

She continued, "I feel like I can breathe again. I've got more space to think, rather than having my parents' needs clawing at me inside my brain."

"That's wonderful," I said. And as I turned to Britney I asked her, "And what about you? What's going through your mind as you listen to what's being said?"

Britney said, "I'm seeing more clearly how I've spent my life getting in and out of abusive relationships. And the realization feels like crap. But, it also feels strong. It's like I've woken up from a dream, and now I can see what's real. What's true. Most of my female relatives spent their lives getting in and out of abusive relationships. Abusive fathers, to abusive boyfriends, to abusive husbands. My mom is finally with a nice guy, though. And I'd like to skip the abusive-husband stage and move straight on to a loving husband."

With tears in her eyes she continued. "I'm so angry about the violence and abuse the women in my family suffered. I talked to my mom about it, and she told me about my aunt. I never met her because my grandparents, my mom's parents, threw her out when she was in her early twenties, just because she stood up to her violent, alcoholic father."

"Fantastic," I said, bringing a surprised gasp or two from the group. "No, I mean that," I assured them, then returned my focus to Britney. "Britney, you have found your rebel aunt."

She smiled through her tears, and the others joined her, recalling the "rebel aunt" from mapping the *Mother-Daughter History Maps* the week before.

"Yes," Britney said. "Mom and I have decided to go and find her. To apologize to her for how she was treated. Mom feels so guilty, because she sided with her parents and didn't stay in touch with her after Grandma and Grandpa made her leave. I tried to tell Mom she was young herself when it all happened. Besides, Mom's not to blame for how her parents behaved. But Mom still feels she should've stopped them."

"The guilt your mom is feeling is called guilt by proxy," I told Britney. "It's the kind of guilt women feel when the perpetrator doesn't take responsibility for the harm he, or she, has caused, and the victim is left feeling all the shame. But you're right about your mom. She's also a victim. She was also harmed by her parents' unwillingness to face the truth of your grandfather's alcoholism and violence. That silence led her to repeat the violence she grew up with in her own life."

"You're going to find your rebel aunt?" Samantha said, turning to Britney. "What a great idea! This is going to be so healing. I really admire what you're doing. You are one strong woman. And I have no doubt that your boyfriend will be out of your life soon, and you won't replace him with another abusive boyfriend. I'm so glad that you have your mom, and hopefully, also a new aunt to get to know. And we have each other." Samantha looked around the circle, then back to Britney. "I'm so glad you came to this group. I wish I had a group like this at your age. I don't think I would've married my husband if I'd had this conversation back then."

Everyone nodded as Britney thanked Samantha.

I would like to pause here and reiterate a point I made earlier in the chapter, that emotionally honest conversations like this do not automatically emerge when women gather in circle. It requires that the facilitator has done her own examination of the sexism she has inherited from her mom, family, and society, and understands the countless ways women silence themselves and each other. The facilitator needs to keep hold of the idea that women are people first, with feelings and needs of their own—and that women's needs *must* have an equal voice in all their relationships.

Without this fundamental rule, women's circles are in danger of repeating the silencing of women. They cannot create a safe environment for women like Danielle to tell the barebones, honest truth about how she feels about her marriage. And the other members would have, in all likelihood, treated her just as they themselves are so often treated. They would have made her feel selfish, that she'd said too much, through their lack of engagement with her needs and emotions. Everyone would have colluded with the emotional silencing of Danielle by redirecting the conversation away from her needs and feelings to what her husband and children need *from* her. And Danielle would have been in great danger of suppressing her newfound voice, and might well have buckled under the pressure she felt from her family to return to her husband for "the good of the family."

Let's return to the circle story and check in with how Samantha is feeling.

I asked Samantha, "How about you? What are you thinking and feeling?"

"I've spent the week with my mother. I had to take her to the hospital for a test," she said.

"I'm so sorry, is she all right?" I asked.

"Well it's been interesting," she said. "There's nothing wrong with her. It all started last Thursday night. She rang at about seven saying she was feeling dizzy, and needed me to come over straightaway. Even though she has access to a nurse in her retirement home, she said she needed me to come because she didn't trust the nurse." She sighed. "Well, that should've been the warning sign, because the nurse wouldn't have pandered to her the way I do. I stayed with her all night, and in the morning I took her to the doctor, who sent her to the hospital for the test. The results came back clear. And now I'm wondering if she made the whole thing up. I've been going over it in my mind, and I'm starting to remember other times she did a similar thing. And every time she did this, I was busy with something else and not giving her my full attention. I had told her that morning that I was going to a painting class, and about our *Women's Power Circle* meeting, and strangely, her dizzy attack came on that evening. A coincidence? I don't think so. I think what happened was that she was afraid my attention was going to be diverted away from her, so she became dizzy with fear."

As she took a breath she said, "Like all of you, something has made me see my life more clearly, and all I see is how I've spent far too much time taking care of people." And as she counted the people out on her fingers she said, "Not one of them has ever offered to support me, not even when I was depressed and in the hospital. Now I'm in my fifties, and I am floundering. I've spent my entire life making sure everyone else is okay and in terms of my life, I'm still at the start. Still where I was at twenty-two, when I left college. I've got a degree from Smith College for goodness' sake. I'm really smart. I... could've done a whole lot more with my life."

She suddenly looked shocked and quickly spluttered, "I'm so sorry. I didn't mean to imply that the years I've spent looking after my kids were unimportant. They are important, but right now I feel so far behind everyone else. I'd never admit this to anyone outside this circle—I know they wouldn't like me for saying it—but I resent my husband's success. I resent that I've loved and supported him, and his success isn't enough of a reward for me. I want to be successful in my own right. And I'm angry that he didn't support me. I feel he let me down."

The response from the group was one I'd seen many times before: sad, knowing nods.

"No," she said after a pause. "I feel he's robbed my time, my energy, and my life. I want the years I've given him back, even though I know I can't have them back." Her voice lowered yet now carried steel. "I know that sounds ungrateful, but that's how I feel. I don't feel that my husband and kids are grateful for all the sacrifices I've made. They don't see it as a sacrifice. They see me as Mom, and moms are supposed to be all giving and caring and not need anything for themselves. They don't see that I could've done something else, that I should've focused more on myself."

A thoughtful silence descended on the circle as each woman considered what Samantha had said, and how they saw themselves reflected in her story. They were each walking in Samantha's shoes, and they well knew those shoes didn't leave a whole lot of space for them to feel, dream, and be supported.

I thanked Samantha for her courage, then said, "First, you don't need to apologize for being honest about what you feel. No woman should have to apologize for speaking her emotional truth. And second, what you're describing is a silent female epidemic, and I know we'll be talking a lot more about this during our six-week circle experience. Countless women hide away the feelings you describe in shame because you're right, the world isn't ready to hear them. But your honesty is so necessary for women today. When women start admitting that they secretly resent their selfless giving, the Culture of Female Service that treats women as the world's caregivers will change. Samantha, you inspire me, you inspire all of us, because you have a huge message to give to the world. Thank you for voicing the silent sadness many women carry in their hearts that they haven't lived their life."

Samantha was glowing as I thanked her. Britney reached out and touched Samantha's arm and said, "Thank you. You've just saved my life. I can see what you're saying in my mother's life, and I don't want to feel like that when I'm fifty."

Danielle and Sandeep together said, "Thank you." Then Sandeep added, "Your courage gives me hope."

Samantha smiled at all of them. "Thank you. One month ago I was having lunch with a good friend of mine, and I told her exactly what I just told you, and she looked shocked. She asked me if I felt guilty. I remember being taken aback by her question: It suggested I should feel guilty. I didn't tell her anything more—at that moment I knew she didn't understand, or didn't want to understand. She's lived her life through her family too, and I guess she's okay with it. But... I felt hurt that she didn't try to understand where I was coming from. She's my oldest and dearest friend."

"You are an uncomfortable mirror for your friend," I said. "She didn't want to see her unlived life in your story. And yes, it is painful when your closest friends reject your truth because it's too hard for them to hear it. You, all of us, are pioneers. We're challenging the generational pattern of women being expected to take too much responsibility for other people's needs, and too little for our own. As women, we're at the cusp of creating a new normal, where saying no and setting our boundaries is no longer selfish or uncaring or uncooperative."

Turning to Samantha, Danielle said, "What about your mom? I totally understand that you need to set boundaries with her, but what about if one day she's telling the truth, that she's really and truly unwell? I would feel so guilty if I hadn't listened to her."

Before Samantha could respond, Sandeep said, "I have the same problem with my mom. But what I'm realizing is that at the end of the day, my life matters too. That it's abusive how my family tries to crowd me out of my own life. I've spent my life taking care of my parents. I've tried to make my mother happy by making up for how my father neglects her. And I'm like Samantha... I'm tired. I'm exhausted and angry, and if I don't do something for myself, I know I'll be sucked into caring for my family for the rest of my life. Know what's even more tragic? I know I make very little difference to how my mother feels. She's unhappy and critical and never thanks me. Why am I neglecting myself when it isn't even making a difference?"

Samantha nodded. "That's exactly what's happening between my mom and me. I can't make her happy. And to answer your question, Danielle, we're paying a lot for my mother's care. There are nurses who can help her. Just because she only wants me, doesn't mean she can always have me. I've made sure that help is there if she needs it, and from now on I'm not going to be at her beck and call. I can't read her mind. I don't always know whether there's something wrong or if she's using illness to control me. All I can do is my best, and as we all know, our best isn't always appreciated."

"You're right," said Danielle in a voice that sounded more as if she was thinking aloud than responding to Samantha.

"These are important points," I said. "We need to ask ourselves: Whose needs are we responsible for, and what do we do when other people's needs clash with ours? Whose needs take precedence? Should Samantha be responsible for her mother's dread of being alone? Should Danielle be responsible for her husband's meeting tonight?"

"And what about Danielle's need to go to this circle meeting? Is her husband responsible for supporting his wife? And why should Sandeep be responsible for her mother's unhappiness, or Britney be responsible for her boyfriend's paranoia he'll be cheated on? Women are socialized to bypass their own needs and go straight to facilitating other people's needs. This has to change. When we bypass our needs we are invisible, and when we're invisible we don't matter."

Again, I would like to pause and affirm that women's circles become life-changing spaces when women's voices and needs are the focus of the conversation. As the maxims in Chapter 8 reveal, women's emotional wellbeing, their equality and visibility in their relationships, demand that women are empowered to ask themselves and each other what they need, and how they can deal with a situation without losing themselves. This is essential in creating families, workplaces, and a world that no longer neglects women. But as Samantha is about to disclose, creating a new normal, where women value their needs with the same degree of intensity that they value their family's needs, is not easy.

"For me, I think there's something very primal behind the pull we feel when someone needs our help," said Samantha. "I don't find it easy to ignore my mother's demands, or anyone's demands for that matter. Last week I realized that I come from a long line of depressed women. My grandmother was depressed, and a highly critical woman. My mom has also been depressed most of her adult life, and she's been taking antidepressants since she was in her thirties, when she had a nervous breakdown. It's never spoken about in the family. I remember my aunt coming over to look after us, and Mom coming home after she'd been gone for two weeks. She spent a lot of time in bed, and we weren't allowed to go upstairs to see her."

Her voice turned childlike. "I really missed her back then. I wanted her to come downstairs and make dinner for us again, and be waiting for me when I got off the school bus. I didn't like my aunt. She was a cold person. She gave us lots of chores to do that Mom used to do for us."

Returning to her normal voice she said, "There's a pattern here. Mom looked after my grandmother until she died, and I'm well on my way to doing the same thing with her. And I've had a nervous breakdown. I was shocked to see in my *Mother-Daughter History Map* how similar Mom's life and mine are. It makes me wonder if Grandma had a breakdown as well."

She stopped speaking for a moment and let out a sigh, but then continued. "Guess it doesn't matter, but Mom was never the same. She became distant and critical like Grandma. And easily overwhelmed. I learned to keep away from her, but I've never stopped wanting her to come back to me, be like she used to be before the breakdown. Maybe that's why I rush over to her home whenever she calls. Maybe I'm still hoping that one day she'll change back into the mom I remember." With a small laugh she said, "Isn't that sad at my age?"

"No," I said, "it's very understandable. We can't switch off our wiring that needs our mom to be there for us. We're hardwired to need a mother who knows and loves us. I'm wondering if the women in your family are extremely bright, and without an outlet for their intelligence they became depressed. Maybe they couldn't cope with the role of financially dependent, all-giving housewife?"

Samantha looked at me, eyes wide. "I think you're right. When I had my breakdown, I couldn't stop crying. I was exhausted. I eventually stopped cooking and cleaning and just...went to bed. I remember my husband being really angry. He used to scream that I was being selfish and neglecting him and the kids. That just made me feel worse. Eventually he packed me off to a psychiatric hospital, and I was put on medication."

"I've managed to get myself off the medication since then, but I can still remember the day I went to the hospital. My husband was talking to Mom, and together they agreed that something had to be done about me. I didn't want to go, but I couldn't fight them. My mom and husband put me in the car and they drove me there. At the time, Mom's lack of support really hurt. Now it feels even more of a betrayal. How could she have done the same thing to me that was done to her? I'm sure no one supported her when she had her breakdown. And no one supported me either, not even her. We were both alone."

Samantha paused to get a tissue to blow her nose and dab her eyes. "I haven't talked about this to anyone because I feel so ashamed. Not even my kids. Last week when we were talking about what we need, I kept thinking back to that time. I couldn't stop wondering why no one in the hospital asked me about how I was feeling about being a mother and wife. They kept saying I needed to get better because my husband and kids need me, they guilt-tripped me into getting better. Looking back, it feels like they only saw me as a wife and mother. I wasn't a person to them. And because my husband was a successful man who didn't beat me, they couldn't understand why I was crying and unable to cope. They couldn't see that I didn't exist. Not in my marriage. Not in life. They couldn't see that my husband's wealth stifled my potential—I couldn't possibly compete with his income. Silly as it sounds, if he hadn't been so successful I might have had more support and more inner desire to go out and claim my dreams and financial independence."

I thanked Samantha for her brave honesty, then asked, "How are you feeling?"

"Relieved. My secret no longer feels so bad." Turning to Sandeep she continued. "It's like you said. I feel as if my mother's demands aren't clawing at my guilt anymore. As if I've stepped back from my story and I see myself in a different light. My mother and I aren't crazy women, like I thought we were. Our breakdowns scream our invisibility. I can't do anything about my Mom's. I can listen to her if I have the energy. But right now, I need to focus on myself. We've all been shaped by neglect, and we've tried to survive by doing what we were told. Now, I see that doing what we're told isn't going to make us feel loved."

Circle Meeting Ends

"That's a wonderful statement on which to close our circle," I said, then looked to the others. "In the last fifteen minutes, I want to go around the circle and ask each of you to share one thing you need to do for yourself this week. Danielle, can we start with you?"

Danielle nodded. "I need to find a good babysitter that I can rely on, so I'm no longer dependent on my husband. I need to stop asking him for support, because he uses it as a weapon to regain control over me."

"Absolutely," I said, and every woman in the room clapped in unison.

"Sandeep, what do you need?" I asked.

"I need to move out of my parents' home."

"Wow," I said. "That's big. What about you, Britney?"

"I need to leave my boyfriend," she said.

"Yeah," everyone chimed in. "Good for you," said Samantha.

"And Samantha, what do you need?" I asked.

"I need to decide when I can visit Mom each week, and stick to that plan."

"This is amazing," I said, nodding as I met each woman's eyes. "I am in total reverence for your strength to speak these needs out loud and have them witnessed by us all. So, by our next meeting, what will you each do to meet these needs? Danielle, what will you do?"

"I'm going to ask around at work to find a babysitter. Someone must know of a schoolgirl or college student who loves children and wants to make some money."

Sandeep cut in. "Danielle, I just had a crazy idea. I'm not sure how big your apartment is, but how about if we talk about me boarding with you. I can't pay much, but I can babysit for you when I don't have classes. I know we only met last week but maybe this could work out for us both."

Everyone was delighted at this turn of events. Danielle's face brightened with hope, and she stood up and hugged Sandeep. "Thank you for suggesting this. Let's talk this week," she said.

"I guess that's what you'll be doing this week," I said to Sandeep.

"Yeah, I guess so," she said with a laugh. "I never dreamed this would've happened tonight. Even if it doesn't work out, having admitted my need to you all has made me feel lighter."

"What about you, Britney?" I asked.

"I'm going to talk to my Mom about how I can leave my boyfriend," she said. "It isn't going to be easy because he can get angry. I don't think I can just leave. I need to do this slowly. And I'm going to ring up my aunts and cousins to see if anyone knows where my aunt is, so Mom and I can visit her."

"Very wise," I said. "It's best to respect your boyfriend's anger and have a plan in place and strong support. Do you have a plan if he becomes violent?"

"No," she said.

"I would feel better if that was part of what you did this week. Hopefully you'll never need it, but if you do, you'll have it in place."

"I understand," she said and nodded.

"And Samantha, what are you going to do this week?" I asked.

"I'm going to buy a diary and plan out my week so I know when I can visit Mom. I know at first I'll probably visit more than I want to. But putting it down in a diary and telling Mom when I can visit is a start."

"I agree," I said. And with these plans in place, I blew out the candle and the circle ended.

AFTERWORD

THE TIME HAS never been more right for women to learn how emotional silence limits their voice and power. Equal rights laws have brought women a long way, but they have not and cannot change women's generational experience of emotional silence and emotional neglect. It is time women uncovered these themes in their lives, and their mother's and grandmother's lives. It is time for women to recognize the dire emotional consequences women face when they surrender their needs in their relationships, families, and workplaces.

I want to emphasize how vital it is that women learn how to listen to themselves and each other. This simple, yet difficult task of listening to what we think, feel, and need is central to healing today's epidemic of mother-daughter conflict, the aggression that is all too common in female relationships, and the rifts in the women's movement. When women fight over who gets to be heard, and whose experience is more valid, women are not standing in their power. They are acting out patriarchy's drama that deflects women's attention away from the sexism that silences them and sets women up for invisibility and conflict.

The truth is, all women deserve to have their reality honored, and there is plenty of space for all women to be heard. I guarantee you that when we listen to all women's truths, women will discover that underneath the obvious differences in our age, race, economic and cultural background, and religious beliefs, we all come from a generational family where women have not been heard enough and not received enough emotional support. We share this common legacy of emotional silence and emotional neglect that is screaming to be understood, healed, and changed. And when we connect with this understanding, divisions and differences melt away. Women gain the emotional entitlement to speak and be heard, and together, women become a powerful force that can no longer be ignored or dismissed.

I've worked with many women in predicaments not unlike the fictional clients in this book, and I applaud them all. These women not only changed their own lives, they changed their daughters' lives, the lives of the women around them, and the ones who will follow them. These women shine a beacon of possibility that all women can speak their deepest truth, without fear of retribution. Based on the outcomes of the thousands of women I've counseled, I find it easy to visualize the outcomes for each character I've used in *The Mother-Daughter Puzzle*. Let's catch up with what they are doing.

Hannah had her baby girl and Ruth and Hannah are enjoying the best years of their relationship. Ruth has let her hair grow long, and replaced her designer suits and dresses with a comfortable pair of jeans. Frank, Ruth's husband, is still angry with Ruth for initiating change, and they hardly speak to each other. A huge difference is that Ruth isn't feeling responsible for Frank's silent anger, as she used to. She knows that the changes she is making are long overdue, and that her marriage problems were created when they got married. She allowed Frank to dictate the terms of their marriage, without realizing it, or understanding the consequences of this. Now, Ruth says, "It's my time and my turn." Hannah too is struggling in her relationship with her father, because he is blaming Hannah for his marital problems. Sadly, Frank's unwillingness to listen to and accommodate his wife's needs is harming the future of his marriage and his relationship with his daughter and granddaughter.

Katherine married her loving boyfriend in a beautiful ceremony. She looked glowing in her off-the-shoulder, white lace, mermaid-style wedding gown. Sadly, Katherine's mother decided to hold tight to her martyrdom. She picked a fight with Katherine the day before the wedding, which gave her the excuse she was looking for to not attend her daughter's wedding. Katherine was deeply hurt by her mother's absence, but like Ruth, she knows that her mother's behavior isn't her fault, or even about her. She understands that her mother couldn't cope with seeing her daughter happy. After a life filled with too much emotional neglect, Katherine's mother has become a bitter woman, emotionally incapable of thinking herself into a more empowered and loving reality.

The last time I saw Isabella she looked like a different person. She had cut her brown hair into a short bob, which framed her round face beautifully. She had graduated from the University of Manchester, England, with a degree in psychology. Isabella's father had reconnected with his long-lost sister, and her mother's sister had left her violent, mentally unstable husband. Isabella's teenage rebellion has saved this family from disintegration and emotional estrangement. They now listen to and inquire after each other's emotional truths, and from what Isabella said, this change probably saved her parents' marriage.

Abigail is enjoying her studies at Oxford University, even though she misses her parents. Miriam is being more emotionally honest with Pontus, her husband, and asking for help when she needs it. And at work, Miriam is learning how to delegate. Every time Miriam and Abigail talk on the phone, or through Skype, they have a ritual of checking in with how they are each feeling, and how they are meeting their emotional needs. The Women's Power Circle Miriam and Abigail started at Abigail's secondary school has grown. It is now being facilitated in other schools in the area, and Miriam is in the process of handing over the coordination of the Women's Power Circles program to a paid manager because the job has become too much for a volunteer.

Samantha's aches and pains are subsiding. She is learning to speak her feelings, rather than rely on her body to speak for her. And in her relationships, especially with her mother and husband, Samantha is learning to not give *great gobs of effort* when the effort is not reciprocated. It is hard, after a lifetime of caregiving, to start focusing on what you need. But Samantha is a determined woman. She is daring herself to rethink how she treats herself and allows herself to be treated. It will be interesting to see how her husband reacts to these changes. Will he resist it like Frank, or embrace it like Isabella's father? And will he recognize that it is fair that after all the years she has sacrificed for him, and their family, that it is now *Samantha's time and Samantha's turn*?

Danielle has filed for divorce. She is putting limits on the negative advice she is willing to listen to from her mother and mother-in-law, and she has emotionally released her soon-to-be ex-husband to his responsibility for his relationship with his children, even if he does not recognize his responsibilities himself. At breakfast each morning, Danielle and Sandeep (who moved in with Danielle because she needed a place to live and Danielle needed help with her children) have created a ritual where they ask each other what emotional needs they have that day, and how they are going to meet them.

Shortly after the circle experience ended, Britney ended her relationship with her paranoid boyfriend. Her mother and circle friends supported her during this time because everyone was concerned about her safety. There were signs that her now ex-boyfriend could be violent when she ended their relationship. Britney and her mother have found Britney's long-lost aunt, and they love spending time with each other. At work, Britney has become more assertive. Sexist remarks no longer scare her into keeping quiet. She now calls them out for what they are.

Tragically, Sandeep's family did not react well to her leaving home. Their anger and accusations that she dishonored the family were terrifying. Her brothers would wait outside her lecture room at college, so as she exited, they could threaten her into returning home. At one point their threats were so alarming, Sandeep had to file a restraining order against her parents and siblings. Sadly, Sandeep's family left her with no choice but to cut all ties with them.

My hope for the future is that all women learn to know that it is human to need. I no longer want to hear women sit in confused silence, in my workshops and classes, when I ask them what their emotional needs are. I want women to know what they need. I want women to enjoy relationships, families, and workplaces where their needs are inquired after and honored. And I hope women will claim their need to gather in circles with their mothers, daughters, and other womenfolk, and together create the conversation that inquires after and honors what women feel, think, need, and desire.

Thank you for reading this book. I hope that it has brought you to a deeper understanding of yourself, and your mother and grandmother, and that it has given you a roadmap on how to be visible in your relationships.

With love and respect,

Rosjke

NOTES

INTRODUCTION

1. Hasseldine, R. (2007). *The Silent Female Scream.* (Nottingham: Women's Bookshelf Publishing), p. 158.
2. My critics are sometimes quick to accuse me of being man hating or man bashing. Why is it man hating or man bashing to tell the truth about how patriarchy and some men have mistreated women? This criticism feels like a deflection against me, and other women, speaking what we know is true. And as this book shows, understanding women's mother-daughter history is vital for women to understand themselves and their relationships, and claim their voice, visibility, and equality.

CHAPTER 2: THE LINK BETWEEN MOTHER-DAUGHTER CONFLICT AND SEXISM

1. See Lily Myers's poem "Shrinking Women" (April 18, 2013). CUPSI13 College National Poetry Slam, Barnard College, New York City, NY. www.youtube.com/watch?v=zQucWXWXp3kwww.buttonpoetry.com
2. See the documentary *Miss Representation*, written, directed, and produced by Jennifer Siebel Newsom, which explores how the media's misrepresentation of women has led to the underrepresentation of women in positions of power. www.missrepresentation.org
3. Rich, A. (1977). *Of Woman Born: Motherhood as Experience and Institution.* (London: Virago), p. 226.
4. Debold, E., Wilson, M., and Malave, I. (1993). *Mother Daughter Revolution: From Betrayal to Power.* (New York: Addison-Wesley), p. 249.
5. Holland, J. (2006). *A Brief History of Misogyny: The World's Oldest Prejudice.* (London: Constable & Robinson), p. 252.

CHAPTER 3: HOW SELFLESS CAREGIVING HARMS THE MOTHER-DAUGHTER RELATIONSHIP

1. Hasseldine, R. (2010). "The Culture of Female Service: Why Do So Many Businesswomen and Entrepreneurs not Have a Robust Sense of their Financial Value?" *Policy Review Magazine* (Issue 7). See other blog articles about The Culture of Female Service at http://www.huffingtonpost.com/author/rosjkehasseldine-267.

CHAPTER 4: A HOLISTIC MODEL THAT STRENGTHENS THE MOTHER-DAUGHTER RELATIONSHIP

1. Caplan, P. J. (2000). *The New Don't Blame Mother: Mending the Mother-Daughter Relationship*. (London: Routledge), pp. 44–45. This book contains a discussion of common mother-blaming myths. Also see Caplan and Hall-McCorquodale (1985).
2. Cochrane, K. (2010). "Why Do So Many Women Have Depression?" *The Guardian*. (April 29).
3. Debold, E., Wilson, M., and Malave, I. (1993). *Mother Daughter Revolution: From Betrayal to Power*. (New York: Addison-Wesley), p. 6.
4. Debold, E., Wilson, M., and Malave, I. (1993). *Mother Daughter Revolution: From Betrayal to Power*. (New York: Addison-Wesley), p. 11.
5. Hasseldine, R. (2007). *The Silent Female Scream*. (Nottingham: Women's Bookshelf Publishing), p. 23.
6. Debold, E., Wilson, M., and Malave, I. (1993). *Mother Daughter Revolution: From Betrayal to Power*. (New York: Addison-Wesley), pp. 17–20.

CHAPTER 7: SPEAKING YOUR TRUTH, CLAIMING YOUR EMOTIONAL NEEDS, AND BEING VISIBLE

1. Hasseldine, R. (2007). *The Silent Female Scream*. (Nottingham: Women's Bookshelf Publishing), p. 69.
2. Hasseldine, R. (2007). *The Silent Female Scream*. (Nottingham: Women's Bookshelf Publishing), p. 166.
3. Hasseldine, R. (2007). *The Silent Female Scream*. (Nottingham: Women's Bookshelf Publishing), pp. 65–72.

CHAPTER 8: CHANGING GENERATIONAL PATTERNS OF SEXISM

1. Dick, K., and Ziering, A. (2016). *The Hunting Ground: The Inside Story of Sexual Assault on American College Campuses*. (New York: Hot Books). For more on the documentary see www.thehuntinggroundfilm.com

BIBLIOGRAPHY

Apter, T. (2004). *You Don't Really Know Me: Why Mothers and Daughters Fight and How Both Can Win*. (New York: W. W. Norton).

Arcana, J. (1981). *Our Mothers' Daughters*. (London: The Women's Press).

Armstrong, S. (2014). *Uprising: A New Age Is Dawning for Every Mother's Daughter*. (New York: Thomas Dunne).

Baker, C. L. and Kline, C. B. (1996). *The Conversation Begins: Mothers and Daughters Talk About Living Feminism*. (New York: Bantam).

Bassoff, E. (1988). *Mothers and Daughters: Loving and Letting Go*. (New York: Plume).

Bassoff, E. (1992). *Mothering Ourselves: Help and Healing for Adult Daughters*. (New York: Plume).

Belenky, M., Clinchy, B., Goldberger, N., and Tarule, J. (1986). *Women's Ways of Knowing: The Development of Self, Voice, and Mind*. (New York: Basic Books).

Bolen, J. S. (2003). *The Millionth Circle: How to Change Ourselves and the World*. (San Francisco: Conari).

Brown, L. M. (1998). *Raising Their Voices: The Politics of Girls' Anger*. (Cambridge: Harvard University Press).

Brown, L. M. (2003). *Girlfighting: Betrayal and Rejection among Girls*. (New York: New York University Press).

Brown, L. M. and Gilligan, C. (1992). *Meeting at the Crossroads: Women's Psychology and Girls' Development*. (Cambridge MA: Harvard University Press).

Buchanan, A. J. (2003). *Mother Shock: Loving Every (Other) Minute of It*. (New York: Seal).

Caplan, P. J. (1981). *Between Women: Lowering the Barriers*. Toronto: Personal Library.

Caplan, P. J. (2000). *The New Don't Blame Mother: Mending the Mother-Daughter Relationship*. (London: Routledge).

Caplan, P. J. and Hall-McCorquodale, I. (1985). "Mother-Blaming in Major Clinical Journals." *American Journal of Orthopsychiatry 55*, pp. 345–353.

Carreck, M. (2002). "The Complex Story of the Mother-Daughter Relationship and its Significance in the Counselling Room." Unpublished M.A. thesis, University of Nottingham.

Chernin, K. (1998). *The Woman who Gave Birth to her Mother*. (New York: Penguin).

Chesler, P. (2001). *Woman's Inhumanity to Woman*. (New York: Nation Books).

Cohen-Sandler, R. and Silver, M. (1999). *I'm Not Mad, I Just Hate You: A New Understanding of Mother-Daughter Conflict*. (New York: Penguin).

Collier, H. V. (1982). *Counseling Women: A Guide for Therapists*. (New York: Macmillan).

Cori, J. L. (2010). *The Emotionally Absent Mother: A Guide to Self-Healing and Getting the Love You Missed*. (New York: The Experiment).

Danticat, E. (1994). *Breath, Eyes, Memory*. (New York: Soho).

Darznik, J. (2011). *The Good Daughter: A Memoir of My Mother's Hidden Life*. (New York: Grand Central).

De Beauvoir, S. (1959). *Memoirs of a Dutiful Daughter*. (London: Penguin).

Debold, E., Wilson, M., and Malave, I. (1993). *Mother Daughter Revolution: From Betrayal to Power*. (New York: Addison-Wesley).

Diamant, A. (1997). *The Red Tent*. (New York: Picador).

Dowling, C. (1981). *The Cinderella Complex: Women's Hidden Fear of Independence*. (New York: Summit).

Edelman, H. (1994). *Motherless Daughters: The Legacy of Loss*. (New York: Bantam).

Edelman, H. (1999). *Mother of My Mother: The Intricate Bond Between Generations*. (New York: Random House).

Eichenbaum, L. and Orbach, S. (1983). *Understanding Women*. (London: Penguin).

Eichenbaum, L. and Orbach, S. (1987). *Between Women: Love, Envy, and Competition in Women's Friendships*. (London: Penguin).

Evans, D. and Evans, S. (2007). *Mother Who? Personal Stories and Insights on Juggling Family, Work, and Life*. (Wavell Heights: Big Sky Publishing).

Fallon, P., Katzman, M., and Wooley, S. (eds). (1994). *Feminist Perspectives on Eating Disorders*. (New York: Guilford).

Feldt, G. (2010). *No Excuses: 9 Ways Women Can Change How We Think About Power*. (Berkeley: Perseus).

Fenchel, G. (1998). *The Mother-Daughter Relationship: Echoes Through Time*. (Northvale NJ: Jason Aronson).

Fingerman, K. (2001). *Aging Mothers and their Adult Daughters: A Study in Mixed Emotions*. (New York: Springer).

Firman, J. and Firman, D. (1989). *Daughters and Mothers: Healing the Relationship*. (New York: Crossroad).

Fischer, L. R. (1986). *Linked Lives: Adult Daughters and their Mothers*. (New York: Harper & Row).

Fox, F. (2003). *Dispatches From a Not-So-Perfect Life: Or How I Learned to Love the House, the Man, the Child.* (New York: Harmony).

French, M. (1987). *Her Mother's Daughter.* (London: Heinemann).

Friday, N. (1977). *My Mother / My Self: The Daughter's Search for Identity.* (New York: Delacorte).

Friedan, B. (1965). *The Feminine Mystique.* (London: Penguin).

Gilligan, C. (1993). *In a Different Voice: Psychological Theory and Women's Development.* (Cambridge: Harvard University Press).

Gilligan, C., Lyons, N., and Hanmer, T. (1990). *Making Connections: The Relational Worlds of Adolescent Girls at Emma Willard School.* (Cambridge: Harvard University Press).

Girls Incorporated of Greater Santa Barbara (1997). *Mother Daughter Choices: A Handbook for the Coordinator.* (Santa Barbara: Advocacy Press).

Gordon, M. (2007). *Circling My Mother.* (New York: Pantheon).

Hamkins, S. and Schultz, R. (2007). *The Mother-Daughter Project: How Mothers and Daughters Can Band Together, Beat the Odds, and Thrive Through Adolescence.* (New York: Penguin).

Hasseldine, R. (2007). "Lifting the Veil on Mothers and Daughters." *The F word.* www.thefword.org.uk/2007/03/uncovering_the-2/

Hasseldine, R. (2007). *The Silent Female Scream.* (Nottingham: Women's Bookshelf Publishing).

Hasseldine, R. (2008). "Why are Women so Critical of Each Other?" *The F word.* www.thefword.org.uk/2008/06/why_are_women_s/

Hasseldine, R. (2010). "The Culture of Female Service: Why Do So Many Businesswomen and Entrepreneurs not Have a Robust Sense of their Financial Value?" *Policy Review Magazine* (Issue 7).

Hasseldine, R. (2015). "Mothers, Daughters and Eating Disorders." *The Huffington Post.* www.huffingtonpost.com/rosjke-hasseldine/mothers-daughters-and-eat_b_6704618.html

Heilbrun, C. (1988). *Writing a Woman's Life.* (New York: Ballantine).

Henry, A. (2004). *Not My Mother's Sister: Generational Conflict and Third-Wave Feminism.* (Bloomington: Indiana University Press).

Holland, J. (2006). *A Brief History of Misogyny: The World's Oldest Prejudice.* (London: Constable & Robinson).

Housden, M. (2004). *Unravelled: The True Story of a Woman Who Dared to Become a Different Kind of Mother.* (London: HarperCollins).

Hurston, Z. (1986). *Their Eyes Were Watching God.* (New York: Virago).

Jong, E. (2000). *What Do Women Want?* (London: Bloomsbury).

Jordan, J., Kaplan, A., Miller, J., Stiver, I., and Surrey, J. (1991). *Women's Growth in Connection: Writings from the Stone Center.* (New York: Guilford).

Kidd, S. M. (2002). *The Dance of the Dissident Daughter: A Woman's Journey from Christian Tradition to the Sacred Feminine.* (New York: HarperCollins).

Kidd, S. M. and Taylor, A. K. (2009). *Traveling with Pomegranates: A Mother-Daughter Story.* (New York: Penguin).

Knapp, C. (2002). *Appetites: Why Women Want.* (Berkeley: Counterpoint).

Knudson-Martin, C., Wells, M., and Samman, S. (eds). (2015). *Socio-Emotional Relationship Therapy: Bridging Emotion, Societal Context, and Couple Interaction.* (London: Springer).

Lawler, S. (2000). *Mothering the Self: Mothers, Daughters, Subjects.* (London: Routledge).

Lerner, H. (1986). *The Dance of Anger: A Woman's Guide to Changing the Patterns of Intimate Relationships.* (New York: Perennial Library).

Lerner, H. (1988). *Women in Therapy.* (New York: Jason Aronson).

Luepnitz, D. (1988). *The Family Interpreted: Feminist Theory in Clinical Practice.* (New York: Basic Books).

Martin, C. (2007). *Perfect Girls, Starving Daughters: How the Quest for Perfection is Harming Young Women.* (New York: Berkley Books).

McBride, K. (2009). *Will I Ever Be Good Enough? Healing the Daughters of Narcissistic Mothers.* (New York: Free Press).

Miller, J. (1986). *Toward a New Psychology of Women.* (Boston: Beacon Press).

Miller, T. (2005). *Making Sense of Motherhood: A Narrative Approach.* (Cambridge: Cambridge University Press).

Moskowitz, F. (ed). (1994). *Her Face in the Mirror: Jewish Women on Mothers and Daughters.* (Boston: Beacon Press).

Myss, C. (1996). *Anatomy of the Spirit: The Seven Stages of Power and Healing.* (New York: Three Rivers Press).

Nafisi, A. (2003). *Reading Lolita in Tehran.* (New York: Random House).

Nafisi, A. (2008). *Things I've Been Silent About: Memories of a Prodigal Daughter.* (London: Random House).

Northrup, C. (2005). *Mother-Daughter Wisdom: Creating a Legacy of Physical and Emotional Health.* (London: Bantam Dell).

O'Reilly, A. (ed). (2004). *Mother Outlaws: Theories and Practices of Empowered Mothering.* (Toronto: Women's Press).

O'Reilly, A. and Abbey, S. (eds). (2000). *Mothers and Daughters: Connection, Empowerment, and Transformation.* (Oxford: Rowman & Littlefield).

Olorenshaw, V. (2016). *Liberating Motherhood: Birthing the Purplestockings Movement.* (Shanagarry: Womancraft Publishing).

Orbach, S. and Eichenbaum, L. (2000). *What Do Women Want?* (London: HarperCollins).

Orenstein, P. (1994). *School Girls: Young Women, Self-Esteem and the Confidence Gap.* (New York: Anchor).

Payne, K. (ed). (1984). *Between Ourselves: Letters Between Mothers and Daughters 1750–1982*. (Boston: Houghton Mifflin).
Pearson, A. (2003). *I Don't Know How She Does It*. (London: Vintage).
Peskowitz, M. (2005). *The Truth Behind the Mommy Wars: Who Decides What Makes a Good Mother?* (Emeryville: Seal).
Phillips, S. (1991). *Beyond the Myths: Mother-Daughter Relationships in Psychology, History, Literature and Everyday Life*. (Sydney: Hampden Press).
Pipher, M. (1994). *Reviving Ophelia: Saving the Selves of Adolescent Girls*. (New York: Grosset/Putnam).
Reynolds, S. and Reynolds, E. (2013). *Mothering & Daughtering: Keeping Your Bond Strong Through the Teen Years*. (Boulder: Sounds True).
Rich, A. (1977). *Of Woman Born: Motherhood as Experience and Institution*. (London: Virago).
Rubin, L. (2000). *Tangled Lives: Daughters, Mothers, and the Crucible of Aging*. (Boston: Beacon Press).
Sandberg, S. (2013). *Lean In: Women, Work, and the Will to Lead*. (New York: Alfred A. Knopf).
Secunda, V. (1992). *When You and Your Mother Can't Be Friends: Resolving the Most Complicated Relationship of Your Life*. (London: Cedar).
Shandler, N. (2002). *Ophelia's Mum: Women Speak Out About Loving and Letting Go of Their Adolescent Daughters*. (London: Vermilion).
Shandler, S. (1999). *Ophelia Speaks: Adolescent Girls Write About Their Search for Self*. (New York: HarperCollins).
Simmons, R. (2002). *Odd Girl Out: The Hidden Culture of Aggression in Girls*. (New York: Harcourt).
Steinem, G. (1983). *Outrageous Acts and Everyday Rebellions*. (New York: Henry Holt).
Straub, G. (2008). *Returning to My Mother's House: Taking Back the Wisdom of the Feminine*. (West Hurley: High Point).
Streep, P. (2009). *Mean Mothers: Overcoming the Legacy of Hurt*. (New York: HarperCollins).
Tannen, D. (2006). *You're Wearing That? Understanding Mothers and Daughters in Conversation*. (New York: Random House).
Taylor, J., Gilligan, C., and Sullivan, A. (1995). *Between Voice and Silence: Women and Girls, Race and Relationship*. (Cambridge: Harvard University Press).
Van Mens-Verhulst, J., Schreurs, K., and Woertman, L. (eds). (1993). *Daughtering and Mothering: Female Subjectivity Reanalysed*. (London: Routledge).
Walker, A. (2005). *In Search of Our Mothers' Gardens: Womanist Prose*. (London: Orion).
Walker, R. (2008). *Baby Love: Choosing Motherhood after a Lifetime of Ambivalence*. (London: Souvenir).
Waterhouse, D. (1997). *Like Mother, Like Daughter: How to Break Free from the Female Food Trap*. (London: HarperCollins).

Wilkinson, R. and Pickett, K. (2009). *The Spirit Level: Why Greater Equality Makes Societies Stronger*. (London: Bloomsbury).

Wiseman, R. (2002). *Queen Bees & Wannabes: Helping Your Daughter Survive Cliques, Gossip, Boyfriends & Other Realities of Adolescence*. (London: Piatkus).

Wolf, N. (2001). *Misconceptions: Truth, Lies, and the Unexpected on the Journey to Motherhood*. (London: Chatto & Windus).

Worrell, J. and Remer, P. (1992). *Feminist Perspectives in Therapy: An Empowerment Model for Women*. (Chichester: John Wiley).

Zoepf, K. (2016). *Excellent Daughters: The Secret Lives of Young Women who are Transforming the Arab World*. (New York: Penguin).

ACKNOWLEDGMENTS

PIONEERING A NEW specialty is not easy. You need a village around you. I am extremely grateful for the people in my village who believe in me and see how needed my mother-daughter work is.

I want to thank the thousands of women, and the occasional man, who had the courage to book an appointment with me. It is a privilege to know you! As I repeatedly say to my clients, mother-daughter therapy and coaching is not for the fainthearted. It takes courage to stand in the truth of your life, and your relationships, and to go against the norms that have silenced and limited you. You have each taught me a great deal about the emotional reality of women's lives, the deeper dynamics of the mother-daughter relationship, and what women need so they feel heard, and I want to thank you for that.

My mother, mother-in-law, grandmother (or Oma as she was called in Dutch), and father (Papa in Dutch) have all passed away. Mom, I know that our relationship was difficult, and I understand that at some level you had little choice about who you were. I truly believe that I was meant to be your daughter, and you were meant to be my mother, because it was through our relationship that I found my passion, this specialty. I will forever be grateful for that. Stella, my mother-in-law, thank you for the times you quietly stood up for me against the angry voices in your family and mine that didn't like what I was saying. I understand how hard that must have been for you. Oma, thank you for showing me that you understood how difficult it was to be my mother's daughter. I feel you around me, encouraging me to speak my truth. I hope that through me, your voice will finally be heard. And Papa, thank you for your unfailing love. I feel your spirit with me all the time. I know that underneath your fear of standing up against my mother's anger, you wanted me to live my life.

John, my partner, soul mate, and love of my life, thank you for your patience, proofreading skills, countless hours of guidance and discussion, and unwavering support. Your belief in my calling to spend my life listening to and studying mothers and daughters has sustained me when I doubted myself, and when the marginalization of this specialization became too much for me. Ben and Olivia, my amazing children, thank you for teaching me about what it means to be your mother, and for your love and support. It is an honor to be your mother.

Lorna Marchant, my supervisor and mentor, thank you for your support and wise counsel, and for the many invigorating conversations we have had. You are a brilliant psychotherapist and supervisor who empowers others to recognize their abilities. Thank you for your nurturing midwifery as I give birth to this new specialty.

My dear friends Antje Bourdages, Deborah Chaze, Saija DiGesu, Vanessa Druskat, Milli Galgut, Teri Hull, Joanne Knight, Susan Newman Manfull, Jennifer Price, Amy Sedgwick, Serena Simmons, Amy Sutley, and others, your love and support means everything to me! I am stronger because you are in my life. Paula Caplan, Serena Simmons, and Amy Sutley, thank you for reading the manuscript and your wise feedback.

Lois Herman, Coordinator of Women's UN Report Network, your support in sharing the message globally is heartwarming. Thank you to all the women who have invited me to speak to their classes, conferences, and organizations, and who pass on my *Huffington Post* blogs and articles to their networks. You are my fellow pioneers. Together we are giving the mother-daughter relationship the recognition it deserves.

And then there are the people who helped create this book. Arlene Robinson, my gifted editor, thank you for your careful editing and helping me polish my words. Ingrid Paulson, my brilliant book designer, I feel honored that you designed this book.

Elizabeth Downing, my life-long web designer, you and I have come a long way together from when you created my first website. I love the conversations we have in between talking about the website. I am so grateful I found you early on in my career. You are a talented artist!

Tim O'Brien, thank you for painting the *Women's Power Circles* and *Mother-Daughter Coach* logo images. I love how you were able to capture so beautifully the work I do. Deborah Chaze, thank you for your lovely photographs. Angela Castrigno, thank you for the amazing video you created for my website. You are all talented artists!

Finally, thanks to all the researchers who have come before me, and I have listed many of you in the bibliography. I feel honored to be standing on your shoulders. You have handed the baton to me, and I hope that through this book, and my training courses, I will pass the baton on to other researchers, counselors, psychotherapists, and coaches.

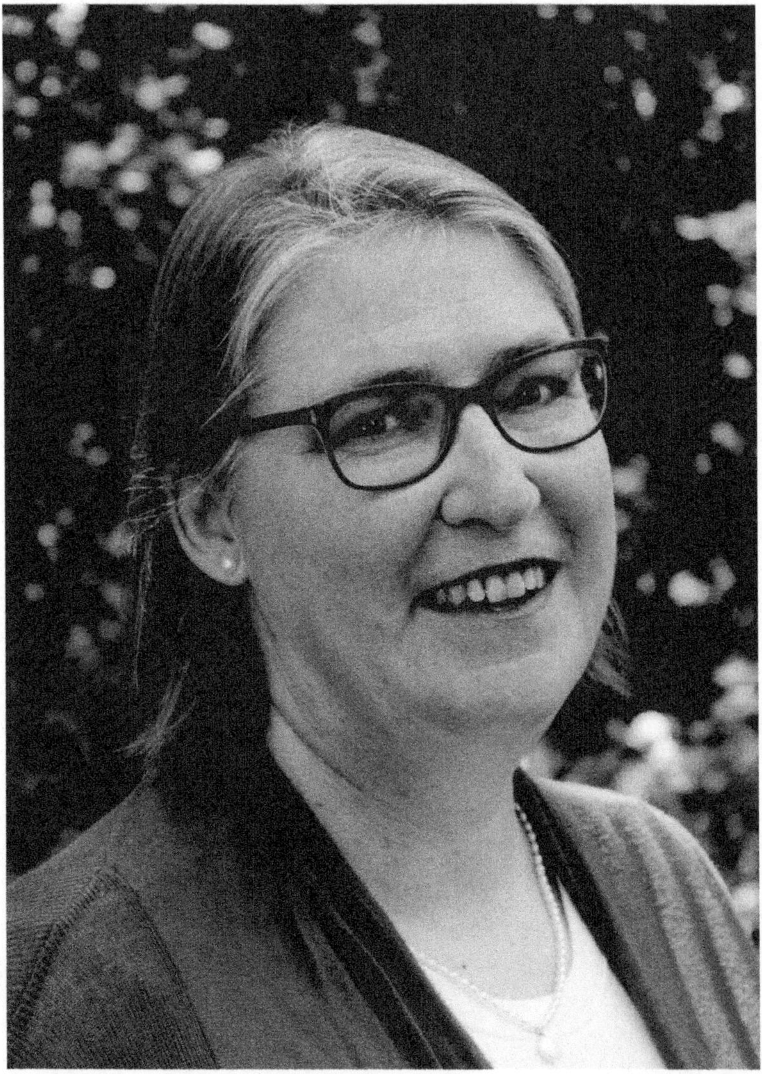

Rosjke Hasseldine, an internationally recognized expert on mother-daughter relationships, has helped thousands of women from around the world heal their mother-daughter relationship. Her first book, *The Silent Female Scream*, aptly detailed the challenges women face in being heard. In *The Mother-Daughter Puzzle* she explains all she has learned through her long career as a mother-daughter relationship therapist/coach, while guiding the reader through her groundbreaking model and *Mother-Daughter History Mapping* exercise.

An accredited and registered psychotherapist with the British Association for Counselling and Psychotherapy, Rosjke holds a master's degree from Indiana University, is a professional member of the American Counseling Association, and recently was a presenter at the 61st Session of the United Nations Commission on the Status of Women. Rosjke has contributed commentary for *BBC Radio*, and been featured in *Psychologies*, *Vice*, *Cosmopolitan*, *She*, *Mother & Baby*, *The Times*, and *The Scotsman*. A native of New Zealand, Rosjke has lived in England, and currently lives in New Hampshire, USA, teaching both her counseling clients and fellow mental health professionals how to uncover the complicated dynamics of the mother-daughter relationship.

Visit **www.rosjke.com**
for more information about
Mother-Daughter Coaching International & Rosjke's
Talks and Workshops · Online Courses
Certified Mother-Daughter Coach Training · Free Articles

Keep connected with Rosjke through
Rosjke's free E-Newsletter
Huffington Post · Twitter @RosjkeH · Facebook · LinkedIn

Join *The Mother-Daughter Puzzle* Facebook group and be part of the conversation that empowers mothers and daughters.

CPSIA information can be obtained
at www.ICGtesting.com
Printed in the USA
BVOW08s1946130617
486807BV00001B/2/P

9 780955 710414